Bodywork

Edgar Unger/Jürgen Rößler

# Bodywork
## POWER FOR WOMEN

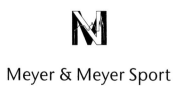

Meyer & Meyer Sport

Original title:
Bodywork – Power für Frauen / Edgar Unger /Jürgen Rößler.
– Aachen : Meyer & Meyer, 1998
Translated by: Anja Haudricourt

British Library Catalouging in Publication Data
A catalogue record for this book is available from the British Library

**Unger, Edgar:**
Bodywork – Power for Women /
Edgar Unger / Jürgen Rößler [Transl.: Anja Haudricourt]
– Oxford: Meyer & Meyer Sport (UK) Ltd., 2000
ISBN 1-84126-022-3

© 2000 by Meyer & Meyer Sport (UK) Ltd
Oxford, Aachen, Olten (CH), Vienna, Québec,
Lansing/Michigan, Adelaide, Auckland, Johannesburg, Budapest
 Member of the World
Sportpublishers Association
Cover photo: Sportfotografie Bongarts, Hamburg
Photos: arena (8/68), Polar (20/28/51/58/67), K2 (70)
Reebok (18/26), all others by Daniel Koch, Büslingen
Cover design: Walter J. Neumann, N&N Design-Studio, Aachen
Cover and Type exposure: frw, Reiner Wahlen, Aachen
Editorial: Dr. Irmgard Jaeger, Aachen, John Coghlan
Typesetting: Stone
Printed and bound in Germany by
Burg Verlag Gastinger GmbH, Stolberg
ISBN 1-84126-022-3
e-mail: verlag@meyer-meyer-sports.com

## CONTENTS

Introduction . . . . . . . . . . . . . . . . . . . . . . . . . . . . . . . . . . . . . . . . . . .7

**I  WHAT WOMEN SHOULD KNOW ABOUT CORRECT
    ORGANISATION OF THEIR TRAINING** . . . . . . . . . . . . . . . . . . . . . . . .**10**

1  Basic Terms of Fitness Training . . . . . . . . . . . . . . . . . . . . . . . . . . . .10
    1.1 A Small Training Theory . . . . . . . . . . . . . . . . . . . . . . . . . . . . . . .10
        1.1.1 Heart and Circulation Training . . . . . . . . . . . . . . . . . . . . . . . .17
        1.1.2 How to Lose Weight – the Principle of Burning Fat . . . . . . . . . .20
        1.1.3 Strength Training . . . . . . . . . . . . . . . . . . . . . . . . . . . . . . . .22
        1.1.4 Agility/Flexibility . . . . . . . . . . . . . . . . . . . . . . . . . . . . . . . .26
        1.1.5 Co-ordination . . . . . . . . . . . . . . . . . . . . . . . . . . . . . . . . . .27
        1.1.6 Speed . . . . . . . . . . . . . . . . . . . . . . . . . . . . . . . . . . . . . . . .27

2  Why Women Should Work-out Differently . . . . . . . . . . . . . . . . . . . . .29
    2.1 Women-specific Training Goals . . . . . . . . . . . . . . . . . . . . . . . . . . .29
    2.2 Bodily Structure/Gender-specific Differences . . . . . . . . . . . . . . . . . .31
    2.3 Specific loads during Day-by-day Routine . . . . . . . . . . . . . . . . . . . . 33
    2.4 Training during and after a Pregnancy . . . . . . . . . . . . . . . . . . . . . .35
    2.5 Osteoporosis . . . . . . . . . . . . . . . . . . . . . . . . . . . . . . . . . . . . . . .37

3  Equipment . . . . . . . . . . . . . . . . . . . . . . . . . . . . . . . . . . . . . . . . . . . .40
    3.1 Outfit . . . . . . . . . . . . . . . . . . . . . . . . . . . . . . . . . . . . . . . . . . . . .40
    3.2 Exercise Gear . . . . . . . . . . . . . . . . . . . . . . . . . . . . . . . . . . . . . . .41
    3.3 The "Mini-studio" within Your Home . . . . . . . . . . . . . . . . . . . . . . .43
    3.4 The Right Choice – how to Find My Fitness Studio . . . . . . . . . . . . . .48
    3.5 Information on Courses offered at Fitness Centres . . . . . . . . . . . . . . .50

4  Nutrition . . . . . . . . . . . . . . . . . . . . . . . . . . . . . . . . . . . . . . . . . . . . .53
    4.1 The Ideal Diet during sporting activity . . . . . . . . . . . . . . . . . . . . . .53
    4.2 Nutritional Supplements . . . . . . . . . . . . . . . . . . . . . . . . . . . . . . . .55
    4.3 Dieting and Fasting . . . . . . . . . . . . . . . . . . . . . . . . . . . . . . . . . . .56

5  Motivation . . . . . . . . . . . . . . . . . . . . . . . . . . . . . . . . . . . . . . . . . . . .59

**II  HOW YOU EXERCISE RIGHT** .................................61

**1  Fitness Test** ...............................................61
   1.1 Endurance ..............................................61
   1.2 Strength ...............................................62
   1.3 Flexibility .............................................65

**2  Exercises** ................................................67
   2.1  Endurance ..............................................67
   2.2  Warm-up ................................................71
   2.3  Stretching .............................................73
   2.4  Gymnastics .............................................80
   2.5  Strengthening with Small Equipment ......................90
      2.5.1  Short Dumb-bells ...................................90
      2.5.2  Therapeutic Band ..................................95
      2.5.3  Pezziball or Fitball ..............................102
   2.6  Work-out in a Fitness Centre ............................105
   2.7  Relaxation .............................................128
   2.8  Basics of Health-oriented Muscle Training ...............129
   2.9  Not like that – Unsuitable Exercises .....................130

**3  Programmes** ...............................................135
   3.1  Beginners All-round Home Programme .....................136
      3.1.1  Without Equipment .................................137
      3.1.2  With the Pezziball ................................136
   3.2  Advanced All-round Home Programme ......................137
      3.2.1  Without Equipment .................................137
      3.2.2  With Short Dumb-bells .............................137
      3.2.3  Short Programme –
         Strenghtening with the Therapeutic Band ...............138
   3.3  Training in a Fitness Centre ............................139
   3.4  Programmes Emphasising Certain Body Parts ................140
      3.4.1  Shoulder-neck-region ..............................140
      3.4.2  Back ..............................................140
      3.4.3  Upper Thighs and Buttock ..........................141
      3.4.4  Abdominals ........................................141

**Appendix** ...................................................142
**Bibliography** ...............................................142

# Introduction

This books wants to motivate you to do something for yourself – for a healthy, beautiful body as well as for your inner balance and your self-confidence. It is devoted to all women, regardless of their age and physical capacity. This book is supposed to help you to take the first hurdle towards a more active life. Nowadays many women suffer from similar problems. Bodily ailments of the support and movement apparatus are overproportionally increasing, the dissatisfaction with one's figure preys heavily on the mind. A lot of people are "drained" from trying to manage the day-to-day problems, as well as handling the increasingly difficult environment.

Usually one tries to improve physical condition in a passive way by taking medicine, testing a new diet or taking powders, capsules and so forth to improve the figure. Most of the time however, only the symptoms can be treated when taking medicine. The success of "slimming-down-products" perhaps is only short-dated – it changes to the opposite all too soon again (jo-jo-effect). The only road to health, productivity, attractiveness and well-being is by being active yourself.

This book wants to give an extensive, easy to understand summary about the topic of fitness training. It is written for beginners, women starting again after a pause, and women with advanced training who want to exercise their body thoughtfully – with, as well as without, work-out gear – to improve their figure.

This book will be a valuable help for coaches as well as exercise-instructors when making an exercise plan, because the exercise developed and chosen in accordance with the latest training, scientific knowledge and health-sport views, almost all can be performed without needing a lot of time. Regardless whether you want to work-out at home, in a club or in a fitness centre, this book will be your guide and companion for the right fitness training.

We all know by now that an adequate physical work-out will prevent you getting sick as easily, slows down the loss of performance and the aging process, and prevents you from being overweight.

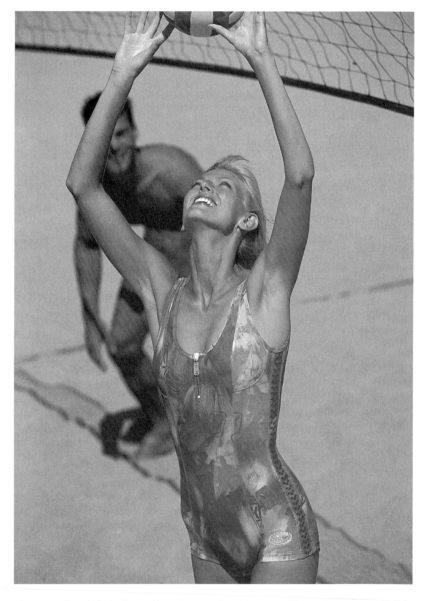

*Figure 1: Closely linked together: fitness – health – joy of living*

It is not simply a matter of proving that regular endurance training does invaluable services for the heart and the circulatory system, or that exercising the muscles of the support and movement apparatus is a preventive as well as a rehabilitative measure regarding backache, arthrotic changes of the joints, osteoporosis, cellulite etc.

Our work-out system takes all of this into account. Above all it improves your muscles, but also takes into consideration the biomotor abilities: endurance and flexibility. The training contents as well as the different exercises selected in this book are strongly oriented on women-specific training goals and muscle regions which are substantial for the prevention of back problems.

Let us motivate you to long-term and regular training by these exercises and programmes which can be performed easily and without having to sacrifice a lot of time.

We would like to thank the owners of the fitness parks TC Kreuzlingen, Lady Fit and Fitln in Konstanz on which premises the pictures were taken as well as the companies Arena and Reebok for the use of their sports equipment.

We would like to put special emphasis on the excellent photographic work of Daniel Koch as well as the committed work of Maarit Schneider, Martina Volz and Uschi Ruckober, who modelled for all the pictures.

# I WHAT WOMEN SHOULD KNOW ABOUT CORRECT ORGANISATION OF THEIR TRAINING

*In principle:* people who are not used doing sports and who are older than 35 years when they want to begin their training should get a physical examination done by a doctor. This applies to all people in this category, even if they feel really healthy. The reason for this is: if there should be unknown injuries of the organs this problem can get worse when exercising. By getting a medical check-up risk-factors can be found which are important with reference to quality and quantity of the training, and which should be considered when making a training programme.

# 1 BASIC TERMS OF FITNESS TRAINING
# 1.1 A Small Training Theory

When the training goal is known from the beginning – for example improvement of the figure, improvement of over-all fitness, or the sport-specific increase of biomotor abilities, it is especially difficult for the sports woman – above all for beginners and those who want to start again after a break – to organise the training units well. The statements of individual coaches as well as of specific literature differ too much. In some sports fields, gyms or fitness centres training forms are being used which have become obsolete a long time ago.

In order to organise the training purposefully and to get the results wanted, the sportswomen or exercise instructors have to thoroughly study the different training options.

The starting point is the term "training stimulus". This stimulus can vary in a lot of ways during training depending on the goal.

**Stimulus intensity:** Intensity of a stimulus. While it is easy to indicate stimulus intensity when working-out or lifting weights by measuring the external force (in kg, kp or even in m/s running speed) it is hard to determine it when playing sport games. If really necessary, only physiological data (lactate, heart rate etc) are helpful as a measuring-source.

**Volume of stimulus:** The volume of the stimulus describes all the individual stimuli of a training unit as a total. In bodybuilding and weightlifting literature it is often calculated as the result of repetitions (stimulus frequency), series and weight (see stimulus intensity) multiplied. So we could calculate the volume of stimulus as follows: 15 repetitions x 3 series x 50 kg = 2,25 tons. Yet there is a mistake in this calculation, because the crucial factor is the respective lifting height of the weight when exercising.

**Stimulus duration:** This can be either the duration of the individual movement or the time span of the exercise series. When using the duration method the duration of the stimulus equals the volume of the stimulus.

**Stimulus density:** The ratio of loading and relaxation time is marked by the kind of rest (full or partly/rewarding) taken.

**Stimulus frequency**: The frequency of stimulus means the volume of loading stimuli within a training unit.

**Training frequency:** As a rule the training frequency is determined by the number of weekly training units.

Whether the chosen activity running, swimming or work-out on machines in a fitness studio, the goal will be set by using the different options – how often, how fast, which weight etc. When co-ordinating the training the reciprocal action of the different options and the sportswomen's shape should be considered. The improvement of shape and prognosis of the biomotor ability "strength" depends – apart from the age and the individual organic and muscular predisposition – especially on a goal-oriented training. By sufficient stimuli the muscle will get tired and energy reserves will be emptied. However, the body tends to keep a dynamic balance between its performance capacity and the demands of the environment. That is why the body, or the muscle, reacts with an over-compensation, which means it fills up its depots above their original levels to increase performance and functionality.

This **over-compensation** is a kind of protective mechanism which is supposed to stop the depots from getting depleted by a repeated load.

To achieve a higher level of performance, by over-compensation, the following principles have to be considered:

- The law of load and recovery.
- The law of progressive overload.
- The law of repetition and continuity.
- The law of individualisation.

After a strenuous muscle training or after work-out on the leg-press, the muscles of the upper thighs are tired and their performance ability is restricted. It is difficult for you to climb stairs or stand up straight from a squatting position. If you would perform the same strenuous training unit for the upper thighs the next day – according to the motto "a lot helps a lot" you will not increase your performance capacity. Quite contraire: some fatigue will remain, you reach the status of overtraining and in the long run this will weaken you because your organism will have no time to refill the depots.

When lifting weights, a beginner needs up to 72 hours to recover; somebody who is used to weight lifting might only need 36 hours. This means that working on the stimulus of specific muscle regions 2-3 times a week is sufficient. But do not wait too long before working on the muscle stimulus again. A work-out only once a week is not enough. The over-compensation gets back to its original level after 3-4 days, so you will not see any results. So much about training frequency.

If the intensity of the work-out is too low, i.e. if you are performing ten repetitions using 20% of your maximum performance capacity, you will not notice any results either because subliminal stimuli do not lead to any adaptation of the organism.

You can keep in mind that correct setting of a stimulus means the best possible harmonisation of volume, intensity and period of recovery. It is necessary to make a long-term training plan of the work-out.

Individual training units which are performed without a plan and only sporadically will not lead to any improvement in training, even when the correct intensity is being used.

Some time or other your body will have got used to the training stimuli which once were so strenuous for you at the beginning. The desired training effect – the improvement of your performance capacity – has been reached. If you want to make further progress, you naturally will have to adjust the above mentioned variables up to the increased level from time to time.

When lifting weights we use the terms sets, series and repetitions. For example, if, in leg-press, you have pushed the machine up ten times without a break that was a set of ten repetitions. It is sufficient for beginners to perform 1-3 sets per exercise, people who are advanced in this activity put up to 3-5 sets.

**Different kinds of muscular tissue:** There are three different kinds of muscular tissue in the body, the **smooth muscles** which can be found in the inner organs such as the digestive system. The smooth muscles contract slowly but with endurance. They are controlled by the vegetative nervous system which we can hardly be influenced at all.

The **cross-striped heart muscle tissue** has to be mentioned, which is controlled by the motor nerves (sinusknot) rather than the conscious will. The heart muscle however can be exercised individually. We will give more details about the sport heart (cardiac hypertrophy) and its advantages in a different chapter of this book.

For bodybuilding the **cross-striped skeletal muscles** are the most important ones. They are controlled by the central nervous system and are able to perform fast and consciously. Skeleton muscles have a beginning (origin), a middle part (belly) and an attachment. The beginning has the more sturdy connection with the bone and is situated closer to the trunk. The attachment is more flexible and further away from the trunk. The origin and the attachment merge into tendons which connect them to the bone and transfer the strength of the muscles to the skeleton.

**Muscle fibre types**: Muscle fibres are determined by heredity and the main loading demands.

**Slower muscle fibres** can be mainly found in muscles with supporting functions, like the musculature of the trunk because continuous stimulation of a low frequency can lead to slow, long lasting contractions. The name of the red muscle fibre comes from the high content of myoglobin. Myoglobin is a substance which helps oxygen to be removed from the blood.

In general, an endurance athlete (i.e. a long-distance runner) has a higher percentage of this type of fibre. In addition to the term red muscle fibre you also will find the names type I or st-fibre ( = slow twitch).

**Fast muscle fibres** predominate in muscles, which mostly have goal-oriented-motoric functions, for example the straightening of the arm (triceps). The content of myoglobin is low. That is the reason why they seem light when looking at them through a microscope. They are therefore called white muscle fibres. These fibres are thicker and have the capacity to develop more strength. In addition to the term white muscle fibre the name type II or ft-fibre ( = fast twitch) is being used.

   The performance limiting factor of the muscle is its ability to tolerate high levels of lactate acid during all high loads between 30 seconds and two minutes. The accumulation of lactate causes an excessive acidity which destroys the cellular milieu in such a way that regular metabolic activity is depleted and the exercise must be discontinued.

**Different adaptability of tonic and phasic muscles:** The common literature mainly uses the following model which should be modified just a little.

Tonic muscles which contain mainly red muscle fibres, in general tend to get shorter. Their main function is to support. The phasic muscles are predominated by white muscles fibres, they have a strong tendency to weaken and are programmed for movement (movement muscles). Due to this, the conclusion was drawn that the tonic muscles should be stretched and the phasic build-up. A lot of muscles do not fit into this pattern. The musculature of the upper back as well as the rear shoulder region, which, without a doubt, has a supportive function and is therefore tonic – tend to weaken and not to shorten – except for a few individual differences.

Differences in adaptability have to be considered when selecting exercises and drawing a work-out plan. Flexor muscles often tend to shorten while extensor muscles tend to weaken. This means that the flexor muscles should be stretched more intensively.

*Among others, the following muscles are among the phasic musculature which have a strong tendency towards weakening:*

- back extensor in the middle thoracic vertebrae
  *(m. longissimus thoracis)*
- rhomboidal muscles
  *(mm. rhomboideii)*
- straight abdominal muscle
  *(m. rectus abdominis)*
- oblique abdominal muscle
  *(m. obliquus externus and internus)*
- gluteal musculature
  *(m. glutaeus maximus and medius)*
- outer part of the knee extensor
  *(m. vastus lateralis)*
- inner part of the knee extensor
  *(m. vastus medialis)*
- saw muscle
  *(m. serratus anterior)*

*These are considered the tonic muscles which take a long time to get fatigued, but they tend to shorten strongly:*

- pectoral muscles
  *(m. pectoralis major)*
- the muscle which lifts the shoulder blade
  *(m. levator scapulae)*
- back extensor in the lumbar vertebrae region
  *(m. erector spinae)*
- hamstring muscles
  *(m. ischiocrurales)*
- hip flexor
  *(m. iliopsoas)*
- short hip flexor
  *(m. adductor brevis)*
- knee extensor
  *(m. rectus femoris)*

We have to take a closer look at the adaptability of some chosen muscles, especially in the trunk, which play a significant role with regard to body-posture. Muscular dysbalance often can causes problems. Most occur in the lumbar and the thoracic spine.

*Mode of Operation of the Skeletal Muscles:*

### a) Static (Isometric) Mode of Operation

During the static mode of operation the angle in which the joints are in does not change, there is no movement. The static mode of operation is used for example to immobilise the shoulder girdle while working at a computer or a typewriter.

Advantages of isometric training are its goal-directed applicability even on small muscle groups, and during short training times the increase of strength is disproportionally high compared with dynamic training loads. It can be used for rehabilitative reasons, when a joint is immobilised and may not be moved. Isometric training does not require any equipment and can be performed without a lot of space; it is therefore ideal to be used during "movement breaks" in an office.

The main disadvantage is the missing co-ordination training, because during the whole training session the joint is fixed in the same position without a functional relation. When doing isometric exercises a lot of people tend to suppress their breathing, meaning they are holding their breath during the loading phase. You can easily recognise if this mistake is being made by the dark red colouring of the face.

### b) Dynamic Mode of Operation

During the dynamic concentric mode of operation the muscle length extends while the tension decreases at the same time. Its function is the acceleration or the active movement of a weight. The advantages are the improved co-ordination of movements during the regular day routine as well as during the sport-specific movements and the improvement of the local muscle endurance. A consistent change between load and unloading is a lot more favourable.

*The five biomotor abilities:*
Five factors strongly determine our performance capacity and our quality of life. For that reason they will be explained in more detail in the next chapter.

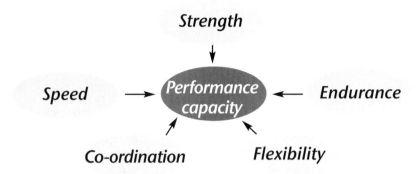

They develop differently during a life-time and can be optimised by appropriate training during the different ages, and can lessen significantly without specific training as one gets older.

### 1.1.1 Heart and Circulation Training

*Endurance* is the ability to keep up a certain performance for as long as possible.

What good does endurance training do? What does such training have to consist of to keep or even improve my health and performance capacity? The following risk factors, divided into internal and external ones, are responsible for developing arteriosclerosis (deposits in the artery) and because of this are causes of a heart attack.

**Internal risk factors**
- Increased cholesterol level
  *(hypercholesterolaemia)*
- Increased blood pressure
  *(hypertension)*
- Increased blood sugar
  *(hyperglycaemia)*
- Increased uric acid level in the blood
  *(hyperuricaemia)*
- Obesity
  *(adipositas)*

**External risk factors**
- Smoking
- Unphysiological nutrition
- Stress
- Lack of movement

### Positive Effects of Endurance Training

All these factors, except for smoking and eating, can be influenced or even improved by a regular endurance training:

- Lowering of the pulse rate in rest and at submaximal loading levels, as well as an extension of the cardiac diastole and hereby an improved blood circulation of the heart.
  A combination of both means economical work of the heart and an improved ratio of demand and usage of oxygen in the heart.

- Lowering of the blood pressure by losing salt as well as weight, respectively decreasing the release of stress hormones (catecholamine).

- Lowering of the cholesterol level, respectively improving the ratio of the harmful LDL and the useful HDL in favour of HDL. LDL (low density lipoprotein) is the main factor for the developement of arteriosclerosis.

- Diabetics can regulate their glucose value into a lower region.

- Usually one underestimates the amount of calories used during endurance training. When running between 30-40 minutes at an average running speed of 6 min/km about 300-400 calories will be used up. In addition to that, the basic metabolic rate will still be elevated hours after the work-out.

- Improved fat-burning (increase of the share of active body mass, see chapter 1.1.2).

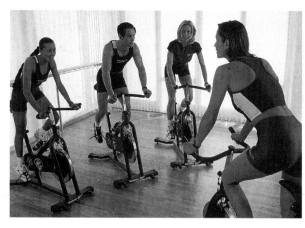

*Figure 2:*
*„Indoor-Cycling" –*
*a new form of*
*endurance training*

## The Four "Golden Rules" of Endurance Training

**1.** At least one sixth of the skeleton musculature should be used when moving, a sixth is the mimimum demand. In general you can say the higher the muscle mass in use is, the more efficent will be the results.

**2.** The duration of the load should not be less than ten minutes to be efficient for the heart circulation system. In order to achieve the above mentioned results on the risk factors, and for an increased fat-acid mobilisation, it should last 30-40 minutes.

**3.** The load intensity depends on age, training and health condition. For correct loading use the rule of thumb: 180 bpm - age = loading pulse rate. Even more general is the advice "trimming 130" which says that during training the heart rate should be at about 130 beats per minute. You can also make proportional indications: the minimum is 50%, the optimum 75% of the maximum heart rate.

The background for this rule of thumb is the knowledge that average persons can reach a pulse rate of about 130 per minute purely aerobicly when doing dynamic sports like running or biking, meaning that the people exercising do not have an oxygen dysbalance. One also speaks about the "steady state" – the use of oxygen equals the intake of oxygen. When increasing the loading intensity, the production of lactate increases as a result of the increasing anaerobical metabolism.

The recommendation: running without puffing is easier to practice in work-outs because no calculation or measuring will be necessary. You should only run so fast that you will still be able to talk to your training partner. Many women who participate in different sports tend to overestimate and overstrain themselves. They run much too fast and by doing this get high pulse rates and therefore risk their health. Heart rate monitors can be a valuable help (see chap. 3.2).

**4.** The optimum of training frequency is four training units a week with about 30-40 minutes . If you can only spare ten minutes, you should work-out daily.

## 1.1.2 How to lose Weight –
### the Principle of Burning Fat

*Rumour:* When intensively train your abdominal muscles you will lose your belly-fat!

Unfortunately this is not the way it works! The body distributes fat-tissue as an energy reservoir, depending on gender, in different parts of the body. Consequently, fat reduction does not work locally. The fat stored last will be used up first in training. There is no doubt that training for the abdominal muscles will tighten the abdominal wall, the love handles has to be worked off in a different way.

*Rumour:* The more intensive you work-out, the faster you improve your figure.

It is certainly correct that you burn-up a lot of calories when moving intensively. Therefore many people try to achieve the maximum in a relatively

## Heart frequency / beats per minute

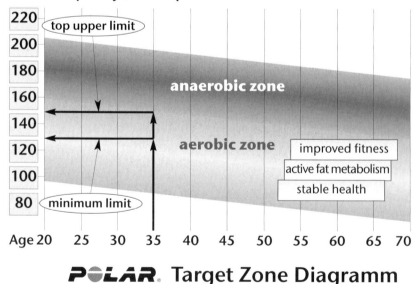

*Figure 3: Diagramm to determine the ideal pulse rate during training*

short time, meaning they put the highest possible load on themselves within the shortest time. Does this really lead to the desired success when trying to get rid of padding?

When increasing load intensity, the lactate production goes up as well as a result of the increasing anaerobic metabolism. Fat can only be burned off under steady-state conditions, meaning the body should be supplied with sufficient amount of oxygen for the corresponding work-out (aerobic load). With this in mind you can tell that it does not make any sense to get to your limit for a short time. Fot the catabolism of fat it is important to do a long-lasting work-out. The more often, and the longer you do sport, the more extensive is the reduction of fat. When reducing your weight, most important is that it is all about using up more calories than intake. That is logical: if the intake is higher, the surplus energy will be stored as fat. You can reach short-lived success with diets or when fasting. When doing so you significantly decrease your calorie intake too. Often you can notice the so called jo-jo-effect however, meaning that shortly after the end of the diet you have put on the weight again.

During drastic fasting-cures, you also lose musculature in addition to water, that is active body mass which mostly will be replaced by fat when putting on weight again. An extremely disadavantageous effect! In addition to that the body switches to its minimum capacity during a diet, the basic "turnover" goes down.

The secret of a good figure lies in a proportional work-out, because it doubles the effect. When doing sport we do not only burn-off calories, but also burn-off fat tissue and build-up muscles. Muscles work like an oven. Even when we do not do anything they use up calories.

How should my training look like to get rid of excess fat at the waist effectively ?
*Very suitable sport activities:* running, cycling, cross-country skiing, rollerblading, rowing, swimming (with limitations, see part II, chapter 2.1).

*Intensity:* about 60% of the maximum performance capacity or the maximum heart rate, respectively.

*Duration:* The longer the work-out, the higher the share of burned fat of the energy used up. A high increase can be indicated after about 30 minutes.

Since the intensity is not very high, the relatively long duration is no problem, the strain load subjectively is within agreeable limits (motto: running without gasping for air). Talking during training should be possible at all times. If you have problems breathing you went beyond your goal.

*Frequency:* Ideal would be for example 3-4 training units of jogging, each lasting 30-40 minutes, per week. Beginners can make walking pauses in between without a problem.

*Result:* You will quickly get closer to your training goal if you reduce the intensity and increase the work-out time.

## 1.1.3 Strength Training

### The Importance of Strength Training for Health

Physical work and use of one's muscles as well as the handling of loads and weights determined the daily routine of the human being for a long time. Many activities have been made easier by mechanisation and automation within a few years. This was a quite positive development when for example thinking about work in industry which was dangerous to one's health. But the people of the western industrial nations now suffer from a lack of basic movement incentives – just think about cars, elevators, escalators and a lot more.

The environment as well as the daily strain have changed a lot, but the human body has stayed the same, it is subject to the biological limits just like it was 100 or 1000 years ago. One of the most important is: "The structure and capacity of an organ is determined by its inheritance and by the quality and quantity of its usage."

A result of our life-style is the drastic increase of the illnesses due to a lack of movement. Contents and goals of fitness training were impressed mainly by analyses of mortality statistics. Nobody paid a lot of attention to the training of the skeletal muscles or their use with reference to health reasons. Scientists put a lot of emphasis on endurance and muscular training which only consider these parameters which play a role with illnesses of the heart circulation system.

Strength training with regard to health reasons is of special importance on orthopedic level. Between the age of 20 and 70, one looses almost half of his skeletal muscles without counteracting this process by muscle training.

Therefore backache has become the most common desease. Rough estimates have shown that about 70% of the German population suffer from backache. A correct muscle training can be recommended from an othopedic as well as medical view as a preventive and also a rehabilitative measure. This is also of importance for children as well as older people.

To make it clear: The function maintains the form, not vice versa. This means that even perfectly developed morphological structures only remain (or improve) if they are being exercised appropriately. When being inactive, these structures will deplete. Starting in-time with a muscle training which is adjusted to one's age and performed regularly and correctly, will strengthen the support and movement apparatus and especially protect the spine by the back muscles.

There is a central importance of strength endurance training in the fitness, leisure and health sports. Strength endurance is the ability of the musculature to keep the movement frequence or posture against longer lasting or repeating static or dynamic demands.

While the maximal strength abilities and especially power abilities play an important role in most sports, our daily strains, for example holding a certain body posture for a longer time, perhaps at a desk, in a car, within the household or at an assembly line, are dominated by strength endurance.

If there is a lack of corresponding training, often muscular imbalance, pain caused by a sedentary life-style, degenerative changes appear. If there is a muscular imbalance, the muscles responsible for the joint are not physiologically balanced.

Shortened muscles have to be stretched, weakened muscles built-up accordingly to get rid of the imbalance. Especially when analysing sitting, it becomes clear that the leg-bending and hip-bending musculature is shortened and that the muscles in the buttock tend to weaken. The result of this is a pelvic position which is very unfavourable for the lumbar spine – and often painful.

In the region of the thoracic spine, and at the shoulder girdle, there are many muscles which tend to weaken, while the chest musculature gets shorter. This leads to the typical round back with a "vulture-neck", breathing problems, head- and backache.

### Strength endurance training

- Intensity: 30-50% of the maximum capacity
- Stimulus duration: 30-60 s
- Sets: 2-5
- Breaks in between the sets: about one minute
- Performance of the movement: slow/medium
- Energy supply: aerobic/anaerobic

The break in between the individual exercises can be shortened as the performance capacity is increasing. People with advanced training experience shorten their breaks by a line-up of the stations (extensor, then flexor). Sometimes the heart rate can be used as a reference level for the length of the breaks. For example: the next exercise can be started when the pulse is below 120.

In addition to exercising strength endurance, the so called muscle build-up training can be used to remove muscular deficits.

## Training to build-up the muscles

- 60-80% of the maximum performance capacity
- 3-5 sets per exercise
- 8-12 repetitions per set
- Incomplete rest (heart rate is at about 120) less than two minutes
- 2-3 stimuli per muscle and week
- 1-2 days rest between the stimuli

For the movement we recommend a rather slow to medium speed. The weights or resistances should be chosen in a way that the musculature used will be totally exhausted and not be able to perform further repetitions after the last repetition without help. Without anticipating the exercise chapter it should be mentioned here that the indications of a maximum performance capacity, or total exhaustion, always include the danger of an overloading, and therefore beginners should avoid such loads. The correct performance of the exercise should be the main thing for people with advanced training experience as well.

## Breathing

In order to perform healthy successful training, it is essential to get used to correct breathing technique. The following general rule is valid for almost all cases:

Your should exhale during the effort, meaning when loading. Explained differently: when you are overcoming the resistance imagine you are exercising your upper body musculature by doing push-ups. Accordingly you inhale when lowering the upper body and exhale when pushing it up.

The mistake which is made most often with breathing during training is the so called press-breathing.

## 1.1.4 Agility/Flexibility

*Flexibility* is the range of movement performed in one or more joints in an arbitrary manner. As a rule the maximum range will be reached between the ages of 11 and 14. A considerable decrease of flexibility starts between the age of 45 and 55 in healthy people.

Causes are the loss of elasticity of the connective tissue as well as the increase of degenerative changes of the joints. Joint stiffness and, resulting from this, a loss of flexibility can considerably reduce your quality of life by influencing your daily routine movements.

Regular (at the best daily) practice, early started flexibility training which takes the most important joints into consideration, will in most cases preserve your flexibility, or even get back some of it. You will find detailed explanations and the most important stretching exercises in chapter 2.3, "Stretching", part II.

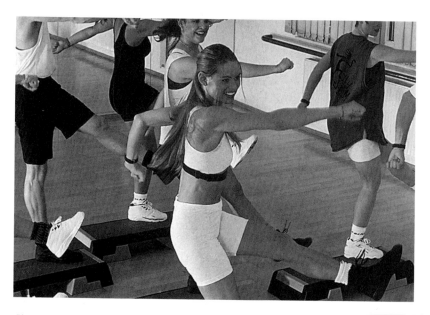

*Figure 4: High demands in reference to co-ordination and flexibility as well are made in step aerobic courses.*

## 1.1.5 Co-ordination

*Co-ordination* is the co-operation of the central nervous system and the skeleton musculature within a certain range of motion. The co-ordination improves, depending on the exercise level, up to the age of 15 or 20. Without specific exercise it constantly decreases after the age of 35-40. A smaller decrease of the fine skillfullness can be found with women when comparing them to men.

When exercising accordingly, you can work against the age-related loss of rough and fine co-ordination which can be proofed by looking at piano-players who, even at a very high age, show a great range of fine co-ordination of the fingers.

The improvement of co-ordination only plays a subordinated role for the prevention of problems with the heart circulation. It is different however during rehabilitation. When co-ordinated well, the demand for oxygen for a given physical performance (for example climbing stairs) can be decreased by up to 20%. This means unloading the work of the heart.

By exercising, meaning the improvement of co-ordination, the movements certainly can be made more economically. On one side the energy and oxygen use gets less. On the other side however the danger of getting injured decreases. 70% of all accidents of old people are due to loss of muscles and impaired co-ordination.

## 1.1.6 Speed

*Speed* describes the maximum tempo one can achieve within a certain time period. When movements are repeated (e.g. 100 m Sprint), speed is called "cyclical speed", within single movements (e.g. tennis service) "acyclical speed". The time duration from any signal to a first muscle reaction is called "reaction speed".

Training speed has a great sport-specific meaning. Its meaning for health is very low however. No increase of the heart circulation system can be reached when exercising speed due to the short time of load.

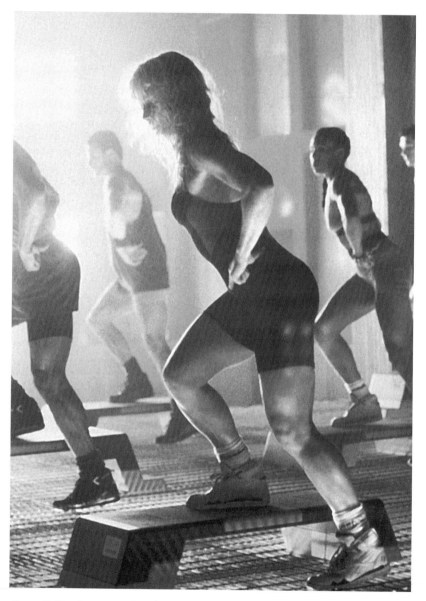

*Figure 5: Step by step getting closer to the goal of tightening the body and burning fat*

# 2 Why Women Should Work-out Differently

## 2.1 Women-specific Training Goals

The interest of women in muscle training is increasing. The quota of females frequenting fitness centres is growing steadily. Some providers are meeting this trend by offering special studios for women only. Just by looking at the work-out equipment one realises that a different way of exercise is offered here.

Concerning the key word "bodybuilding" we must give an explanation. Working out with dumb-bells or on work-out equipment does not automatically mean huge piles of muscles and broad shoulders. The male sex hormone testosterone is responsible for these symptoms.

Bodybuilders, as reported by the media, arouse the suspicion that these results have been achieved by the increased intake of hormones. Even then, a very special high intensity training pattern is needed.

Bodyforming, bodystyling or bodyshaping – whatever the trends in the fitness market are called – the main prospect is to get in better shape and to get a better figure by exercising with or against the resistance of dumb-bells, work-out gear and machines. It is important to know that you cannot lose weight due to muscle training only. Working out increases the percentage of muscles in the body, and muscles have a higher specific weight than fat tissue.

So the work-out results cannot be checked by simply looking at the scale. The muscles as well as the tissue of the individual body parts will be tightened. You get this result by using light weights and performing high repetitions.

As explained before, the body deposits calories which are not burned up – depending on the gender – in certain parts of the body. For women these parts are mainly buttocks and thighs, the lower belly section, bosom and sometimes the back of the upper arm.

*inflammation*
*NOT*

This has lead to the ugly word "problem zones". Cellulitis is a specific prob-lem for women because women, contrary to men, often suffer from weak connective tissue. Additionally the subcutaneous fat tissue in the hip- and thigh region is developed much stronger because of genetic reasons.

Cellulitis certainly is not an illness but rather a sign of lack of exercise and malnutrition. The beginning of cellulitis is characterised by the collection of fat and water in the particular body parts. Only special exercise for the muscles on a regular basis – combined with a low salt and fat diet aimed at dehydrating the body – can bring tight tissue, prevent the develope-ment of cellulitis, or at least reduce it.

Especially recommended is (under) water gymnastics because the work-out against the resistance of the water is an ideal exercise to increase strength endurance. When performing this work-out, one additionally ex-periences the "side effect" of a tightening of the extremities involved.

A nicer figure, and a more trained body, do not just increase self-confi-dence but also increase your overall strength on a day-to-day basis.

Painful neck or shoulder strains are unpleasant associated symptoms to the professional work-load – especially for women who work at a desk or on a computer. But the day-to-day household-chores also can cause shoul-der as well as neck problems.

In addition, psychological problems or stress-filled situations can increase the strain on these body regions contrary to men. Therefore another exercise goal is the strenghtening and stretching of the neck and shoulder muscles.

Even while pregnant there are specific exercise recommendations to obey (see chapter 2.4). Scientists have not come to a mutual agreement concern-ing the exact numbers but they did agree on the subject itself. Exercise re-duces the risk of getting breast cancer. Statistically some tests point to a risk reduction of 37%, others even to a 72% lower risk of getting breast cancer.

It should not be denied however, that, especially for girls, intensive sports-related endurance work can lead to disorders of the hormone system. The possible consequences are: a delayed start of puberty, trouble with the menstrual cycle or even a complete cessation. It therefore seems very reasonable to start intensive training after the first menarche or give preference to the health-oriented training exercises.

## 2.2 Body Structure/Gender-specific Differences

On the average, woman are 10 cm shorter and 10 to 20 kg lighter than men. The amount of fat in a woman's body amounts to approx. 30% (in men approx. 20%) of the body mass. The total amount of blood in women is less than in men, the exercise pulse is higher compared to men's due to the smaller heart volume.

In comparison with a woman's total body weight, whose share of muscles amounts to about 25-35%, men have 40-45%. The extremities make up the main difference while only insignificant differences can be noticed in the trunk. When taking an average of all muscle groups the maximum strength of a woman amounts to only 70% of that of a man. This is due mainly to the tissue-building effect of the male sex hormone (testosterone). The proportional increase of the strength abilities due to training is the same for men and women.

In women the muscles of the lower extremities respond to a work-out a lot more strongly than those of the upper extremities. A man's muscles of the upper thighs decrease (atrophy) because of age or inactivity faster than the arm or shoulder muscles do. Yet when making statements like this, it should always be kept in mind that there are individual genetic differences as well as exceptions to the rule.

If the different upbringing of infants and toddlers with regard to their gender plays a rule in developing the strength abilities this cannot be discussed here due to a lack of research in this area. It is a fact however, that boys are asked to show and develop their "strength" all the time – something that is totally neglected when raising girls. Looking at it from a traditional point of view, having powerful muscles never was a desirable goal for women. During the early years the positive effect of a regular, general muscle training on the minerals in the bones was recognised and was used to prevent and treat osteoporosis.

Looking at it from a sports-medical point of view, there is no necessity not to train during menstruation. Of course there is a rumour that women are less efficient during their menstrual cycle. But all the examinations have shown that about 70% of all women are equally or even more productive at this time. The first half of the cycle up to ovulation is regarded as the more efficient phase, during which all forms of training – even very intensive – are possible. After ovulation the load should be eased a little. In addition, one can show that women who do not participate in any sport activities complain about menstrual problems more often than those who regularly do sport.

Often a combination of light training and relaxing exercises help to prevent menstrual syndromes like headaches, depression or lack of motivation. Here it is recommended to do back and abdominal gymnastics, self-organised training, stretching as well as visiting the sauna.

### Should you do sport even though your nose is running?

Especially in autumn and winter you ask yourself whether it makes sense to pause or to continue your sport activities on a smaller basis, while you are having a cold. All doctors are in agreement that a complete pause from sport must be taken when running a fever and/or having an infection, influenza or cold. This also is valid for the first three days after the fever is down. Most mistakes are made especially during this time because once the body temperature is back to normal most athletes become active right away to make up for the lost training and the loss in performance. This often results in a relapse, not being allowed to do any sports and an even longer pause. Having a fever always should be taken very seriously because combined with sport activities an infection can lead to an acute inflammation of the heart muscle, a damage which often will not be recognised until later. After getting a 'flu-shot sportswomen should decrease their activities for 5-7 days as well.

Having a cold without running a fever however is no reason to stop participating in sport activities. *Very important* is a good hydration now, meaning a sufficient supply of fluids during sport and perhaps prefering warm tea over cold thirst quenchers.

*By the way:* It has been proved that sport has a stimulating effect on the body's power of resistance. The reason top-athletes are more prone to get infections is that their body is being put under a lot more strain – up to the limit – which leads to a debilitation of the immune system.

## 2.3 Specific Loads during Day-by-day Routine

Many women-specific physical pressures of the ordinary day routines have negative effects on the axis organ, meaning the spine. Sitting at a desk or in front of a computer puts heavy strains on the shoulder/neck region if re-peated as does one-sided carrying at home (small children, groceries). Furthermore, a lot of activities in the household are known for their uner-gonomical designed work areas, bending-forward movements are quite common but increase tenseness.

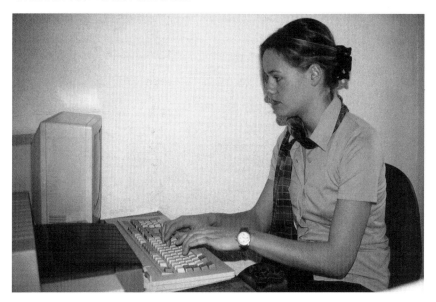

*Figure 6:   Tenseness and backache as a result of ill-balanced strain in day-by-day situations*

Why are these strains so bad for the back? When sitting up straight, there is an axial strain on the spine, therefore the pressure is balanced-out evenly. When bending this lowers the load tolerance greatly. As an example, we can look at a pencil which does not get destroyed when standing it up straight but does when under the pressure of being bent. Furthermore, a crooked posture narrows down the chest and belly areas which results in a limitation of the function of the inner organs and a shortening of the front trunk muscles.

How can incorrect strains be avoided or at least be reduced?

For an upright posture the pelvis has to be pushed forward, the thoracic cage lifted and the cervical vertebrae straightened. Whether in schools, buses, cars and offices we sit on chairs which prevent an upright posture. The seats should be slightly angled forward for an easy tipping of the pelvis and they should have a back-rest bent backwards to support the lumbar region which lifts up the thoracic cage. The spine of the cervical vertebrae is stretched, the chin pulled back towards the throat. The legs should be in a 90° angle when looking at them from above over the knees and feet.

Sitting on so called balancing-chairs which have a support for the knees does help to keep the back straight but in the long run it leads to a shortening of the adductors and the hip and leg muscles – for that reason it is not really recommended.

Among other things participants of "back" schools are taught how to sit on big gymnastic balls. These balls have the great advantage of encouraging the people to sit actively. One automatically moves up and down, back and forth. By doing this, the moving impulses are moved onto the muscles of the back which is good for them.

The ball has to be pumped-up enough for the buttock of the person sitting on it to be slightly higher than the knee so the foward-tipping of the pelvis is easier. You have to pay attention to a straight-up position and the tightening of the shoulder blades yourself however, the ball does not do that for you.

But the gymnastic ball only is a temporary alternative to chairs which support the back, because "sitting actively" is a kind of muscle training that should not be overdone. When sitting on a gymnastic ball for a while, the hold and support muscles will get fatigue as the sitting position is anything but supporting then.

When standing, the body weight has to be divided evenly on both feet, the feet slightly pointing outwards. The thoracic cage should be straight and the pelvis should be tipped forward a little.

When bending or lifting, people often neglect to bend their knees. Bent knees are the basic precondition for a straight back while bending. The feet are pointed outwards and are spread further apart than the hips. The pelvic bone is tipped forward, the thorax straightened, the shoulders slightly pulled back. The buttock should be held up relatively high while bending.

If this position can be held when picking up something, there will not be a wrong loading of the vertebra discs.

The adductors and the hip and leg muscles of most people living in the western industrial countries are shortened so much that they are only able to pick up a stool this way at the very most.

When picking up things which are lying on the ground, these people have to go down to the ground with one knee in order to keep the back straight. When bending or lifting up things you also have to keep in mind not to work outside of the trunk sector. The trunk sector is restricted by the 90° position of the knees.

## 2.4  Training during and after a Pregnancy

Often women who are actively doing sports are insecure once they are pregnant. What am I allowed to do, what not? What can be harmful for the pregnant woman, what can be of harm for the foetus? In order to do nothing wrong at all a lot of people are overprotective. From a medical as well as a psychological view this is a mistake. Also starting to exercise again after giving birth is easier after only a short pause. The latest examinations are even showing an increase of performance during a pregnancy.

The maximum intake of oxygen increases, the production of lactate when stepping over the aerobic/anaerobic threshold is lower and the heart rate does not go up as fast when being under this pressure.

Nevertheless, when participating in sport activities during a pregnancy, one should take into consideration the following aspects:

**Medical check-up**: If there are no complications, the pregnant woman can do sports until shortly before giving birth. Yet the first twelve weeks are a rather sensitive phase; any kind of vibrations should be avoided. Ideal during this time is swimming, best of all backstroke.

**Avoid falling:** It is wise to give up skating, downhill skiing (if at all, ski on flat slopes), soccer, volleyball and handball. Due to the change of hormones, ligaments and tendons will loosen up which results in a loss of stability, therefore the risk of getting injured during a pregnancy increases anyway. You should be more careful when working-out, preferring well-controlled endurance sports like swimming (no breast stroke swimming, swim crawl and backstroke instead), walking, cycling.

**Intensity:** In order to avoid strong concussions on one side and not to let the body temperature rise too much on the other you must keep in mind not to let the pulse rise to above 140 beats/minute and later-on reduce it to 130. If you want to slow down a rising temperature, you have to follow this rule: drink a lot during and after training. It is not adviseable to participate in competitions, especially during the last third of the pregnancy.

**What to watch for when doing fitness and strengthening work-out:**
Generally the resistance should be lowered and the volume of repetitions increased instead. Or even better, switch from intensive strengthening exercises with equipment and dumb-bells to softly strengthening gymnastics, perhaps with a Therapeutic Band (an expanding exercise band) and stretching. Reduce the work on the abdominal muscles or stop it completely, but start up with it intensively after giving birth (exception: caesarean section).

While being pregnant, you should restrain yourself from any exercises you have to do while lying on your back. It is recommended, with regard to the exercises after giving birth, an increased holding and carrying effort in the shoulder and arm region to strengthen the upper back area as well as the arm and chest muscles. Include loosening-up exercises for the shoulder section to loosen up tenseness.

Working the pelvic muscles should be a part of your training plan during, as well as after, the pregnany. The ideal training tool during and also after a pregnancy is the Pezzi- or Fitball (a big and light plastic ball). When doing strengthening exercises, the emphasis should be put on strengthening and stretching exercises for the trunk musculature. Getting a hollow back during pregnancy, as well as the lifting and holding burden after birth, can lead to problems with the back.

Since women tend to strong mood changes during and after pregnancy due to the hormone readjustment there should be a lot of relaxation time during training – this should consciously be planned beforehand. Hot and cold showers for example, or massages for the belly and legs with a brush are helpful.

Right after giving birth one can do light gymnastics. 6-8 weeks after birth the training routine can be started up again. The longer the break lasts, the harder it will be to work-off unnecessary subcutaneous layers of fat. Mothers who are breast-feeding should not put too much strain on themselves during the work-out: 50% of the strength capacity and about 60-70% of the maximum heart circulation capacity are enough to start up again. Endurance training on the exercise bike, tread mill or stepper prevent the developing of varicose veins.

# 2.5 Osteoporosis

Osteoporosis (softening of the bone) is an aging process of the bones which should be taken very seriously. Women mainly are effected by it after the change of hormones during the menopause. An imbalance of the build-up and the demolition of the bone reduces the density of the bone.

The bone trabeculae which are of great importance decrease, the (bone) skeleton loses about 2-5% of its mass each year, meaning that the bone becomes brittle and breaks easier. When having osteoporosis in an advanced stage small incidents or accidents can lead to very serious injuries (fractures).

Especially at risk are the body of vertebrals, the neck of femur, and the lower arm. Physical therapy, nutrition and hormone therapy are the three pillars of osteoporosis treatment.

Hormone therapy at the beginning of the menopause makes sense in a lot of cases but unwanted sideeffects are highly possible which makes medical care unavoidable.

With osteoporosis the bone loses minerals, especially the important element calcium – without calcium the build-up of bones would be impossible. For preventative as well as therapeutic reasons one should therefore make sure to have a diet rich in calcium which is found in milk products, fish, vegetables (i.e. broccoli). Calcium in the form of patent medicine can be substituted.

Especially damaging to the blood vessels, which are especially tiny in bones, is smoking and therefore this facilitates the development of osteoporosis.

For more than only one reason exercising is the ideal precaution as well as therapy. More than once it has been proved in scientific work that the bone structure is defined by the mechanical power of pressure. During a well-proportioned and detailed muscle training, the bones are subject to pull as well as pressure strain. This increases the activity of the bone-building cells, more calcium is stored and the bone trabeculae move accordingly. Of course the muscle training should be performed around the axis so there will not be any bending tensions.

Since an active muscle – similar to the heart – works like a blood pump, muscle training improves the blood circulation of the corresponding body part, and therefore provides a better supply to the bones. An analysis about the subject "density of the bones in relation to physical activity" proved, that endurance training has a positive effect. When working out with weights the results were even better, but most effective for the prevention of osteoporosis was combined strength and endurance work.

This becomes very clear when looking at the negative example of astronauts. Because of the lack of gravity the body hardly performs any work at all, the musculature loses tone and the bone capacity is significantly reduced after a long stay in space.

A further positive effect of sport activities is that your co-ordination improves. Sudden falls cannot be as bad even when the bones are "not perfect anymore" – you simply fall more skillfully or not at all.

# 3 Equipment

## 3.1 Outfit

Here rather functional than fashionable aspects should be considered. Even though the sport clothing industry tries to tell us that special outfits are needed for each individual sport trend, there is no reason why you cannot play streetball or go bungee-jumping in a regular sweat shirt and cotton shorts or jogging pants. You should not overlook that you should "feel comfortable" when doing sport. And for that purpose you need the right clothing. Those who want to show-off their special taste will certainly find something in the broad range of sport fashion offered. In some sport studios you will notice a trend towards a certain fashion. Either you go along, change the studio or you purposely swim against the "fashion" tide. Regardless of your decision do not forget that having fun is very important, too.

With some sport activities, for example jogging, it makes sense to attach importance to special equipment (i.e. functional jogging shoes).

The "onion-principle" is recommended for many outdoor activities (jogging, cycling, mountain biking, hiking etc). Various peaces of clothing for different purposes worn on top of each other provide a fast and flexible adjustment to changing weather conditions. The layer (of clothes) closest to the skin should consist of sweat-transporting artifical fibre in order to prevent the skins' cool-off by evaporation.

Above this you should best wear a material which keeps the warmth inside, stores the sweat, or ideally transfer it. The top layer should consist of wind and water-resisting material, which should actively breath (i.e. Gore-tex). Although the advertisements promise a lot, many of their promises turn out to be not true in reality. There is no need for you to create a climate as in a sauna.

A lot of women think that detailed muscle training is good for the breast and that the breast will get a "lift" when strengthening the breast muscles. Without a doubt specific training for the shoulders (especially strengthening of the upper back region and stretching of the breast muscles) leads to an improved, more straight body position in the upper trunk area, which also leads to a lift of the breast. We have written about the tightening of the connective tissue in an earlier section of this book. However we cannot speak about a systematic training of the breast since it does not consist of muscles but a combination of glands and fat tissue. When doing sport it is important for the breast to get a supportive steadiness because an ill-fitting bra, or wearing none, can put too much strain on the connective tissue; any kind of movement will feel "disturbing". There is a broad variety of bra models and you will find the right one for each size and activity.

**What do I have to consider when buying a bra?**
- Optimum support of the breast, tight fit without being constricting.
- Comfortable wear because of soft, seamless cups and otherwise flat seams.
- Fabric which does not rub on the skin and which is light and elastic.
- A cut which leaves room to move and possibly stays off the shoulder blades.
- Secure support of the straps.
- Hooks which will not cause any injuries to the back.

# 3.2 Exercise Gear

For the most important kinds of endurance sport, working-out in gymnastic groups or in studios there is no need to buy expensive equipment (at the most jogging shoes, bike).

Recommended for training in a studio: sport shoes with a solid sole, training gloves to avoid calluses on the hands, comfortable, elastic, sweat-absorbing clothes which will not limit your freedom of movement, and a towel, should be mandatory. For the wet cells we recommend bathing slippers and for the sauna visit two big towels and perhaps a bathrobe.

Ambitious endurance athletes meanwhile are able to buy reasonably priced machines to diagnose their capacities and direct their training which in former times was only available, if at all, in professional sponsored sports.

The easiest way for the correct training doses is to control the heart rate. Certainly this can be done by checking your pulse (wrist or throat next to the larynx) with a clock, but to do this training has to be interrupted. If the pulse beat is not found right away the measurement is not accurate since the pulse can go down again very quickly. It is easier and more accurate to measure the heart rate with a heart rate monitor.

The heart rate monitor wich are easy to use can be bought in special stores from approx. £ 45 UK/$ 70 US/$ 100 Cdn up. They consist of a belt for the chest with a built-in transmitter and a wristwatch which evaluates the current heart rate and indicates it. The lower and the upper limit of the ideal training can be programmed in, and the gadget will start bleeping once you are over or under these rates telling you whether to reduce or increase the load.

An important value to determine your capacity is the recovery pulse rate because a well-trained heart circulation system goes back to its starting point after a work-out faster than an untrained one. Therefore you should check the heart rate again 3-5 minutes after the end of training and compare these values over a longer training period.

More precise, but more time-consuming and more expensive as well is checking the lactate level. The value control lactate is measured in millimol per litre blood and should not be over 4 mMol during methodical fitness training. Ideal for the aerobic endurance training would be between 2 and 4 mMol.

The lactate analyser by Accusport can be bought for about £ 200 UK/ $ 330 US/$ 480 Cdn up in special stores and can be used to randomly check the lactate level when training, or to determine the ideal goal setting by performing a graded test.

By measuring the heart rate and the lactate level at the same time you can accurately determine the transition from the aerobic to the anaerobic level. The ideal heart rate for endurance training can be determined more individually than with a regular formular provided that there is a step by step increase of the load on the tread mill or the exercise bike. For this you prick a drop of blood out of the earlobe or the finger tip, put it on a measuring strip which, – with the help of tiny measuring equipment, will show the accurate lactate level within a short time frame.

## 3.3 The "Mini-studio" within Your Home

There is no doubt that the easiest way to keep in shape is the regular visit to a fitness centre or to join a training group in a sports club. The people who do not like either one of these options can stay fit at home as well.

But one should have some knowledge about the planning of training and its content because neither a coach, nor an exercise instructor, will be by your side at home to watch if you perform the exercises correctly.

You do not have to get an expensive, space-consuming multifunctional set-up for your living room. With the help of some inexpensive apparatus which will not take up a lot of room you can perform a diversified and significant training.

But you should think about your training objective and which equipment you need to reach your goals best before buying anything.

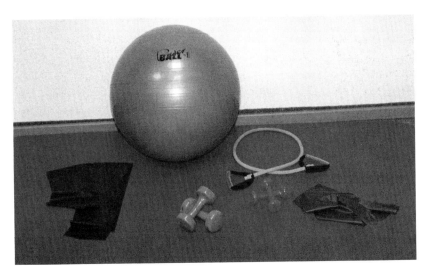

*Figure 7: Inexpensive and not using up a lot of room: equipment for training at home*

## Skipping Rope

A cheap classic! It cannot really be beaten when doing cost-use amount of space needed comparisons. After a short time you will get the hang of it and challenges will give a further incentive. This sport is considerate to your neighbours as well as to your joints if you use a soft mat or carpet, or well-absorbing sport-shoes.

*Training focus:* Excellent for endurance and co-ordination

*Price:* Starting at £ 3 UK/$ 5 US/$ 7 Cdn up with ergonomical grips, ball-bearings and leather rope starting at £ 12 UK/$ 20 US/$ 27 Cdn up

## Mini Trampoline

Before buying one should check the height of the ceiling to avoid an unpleasant surprise. It is a gentle training apparatus because it is easy on the joints and the strain on the heart circulation system can be controlled. Diversified training by using different jumping techniques: alternated hops, two-footed jumps with knee lift, two-footed jumps with legs straddled, hops on one leg. Here the same should be considered as with the skipping rope: if you use a soft support (i.e. carpet, gymnastic mat) you will not get on your neighbour's nerves.

*Training focus:* Good for endurance, co-ordination and balance.

*Price:* Starting at £ 30 UK/$ 47 US/$ 70 Cdn up.

## Pezzi- or Fitball

We have to get rid of one presumption right away: the Pezziball or Fitball is a training tool and not a piece of furniture to sit on. It can be used in an office or in front of the TV but only as a temporary alternative because, just like with every other exercise, the same rule applies here. It is the right amount of exercise which brings success. People who switch their office chair just for one day with the Fitball to do their back some good should not be surprised if the back musculature is stiff or sore the next day, just like after a work-out. By sitting actively the lower back muscles, the leg muscles and the feeling for balance, will be exercised softly without doing a special exercise for it. But furthermore, there are a lot of special abdominals, back and leg exercises which are also helpful to the spine which you can do with the ball. Watch for the right size! When sitting on the ball, the upper thighs should be pointed slightly downwards.

*Training focus:* Co-ordination and strengthening

*Price:* Starting at £ 10 UK/$ 15 US/$ 20 Cdn up

**Therapeutic Band**
The good old expander is no longer in use! Limited when it came to exercise variations and measurement and not really ideal with regard to the distribution of strength during an exercise, this classic had to make room for the Therapeutic Band. As well as through the range of bands in different tightnesses, as by the possibility of folding the bands repeatedly, this training tool can be adjusted perfectly to the different exercise needs and objectives. Different grips, clips to make loops (making knots also is okay) and textile loops to fasten it to the door give you numerous exercise forms (also look at the exercise part of this book). Because it uses up so little room the thera band is an ideal training companion when travelling as well.

*Training focus:* Strengthening

*Price:* Starting at £ 5 UK/$ 7 US/$ 10 Cdn up (often available by the metre, ideal 1,5-2 m length, often a poster with exercise ideas is enclosed). As a set with grips and bands of different strengths: starting at £ 7 UK/$ 3,50 US/$ 17 Cdn up.

**Feather Grips**
Very limited training tool which can be stored well however in the drawer of a desk or a computer work place to "exercise your fingers" from time to time. Otherwise used mainly for specific sports (climbing, tennis, squash, badminton etc).

*Training focus:* Strengthening hands and fingers

*Price:* Starting at £ 2,50 UK/$ 4 US/$ 5 Cdn up.

**Short Dumb-bells**
You can perform a strengthening programme for shoulder, chest and arms by using several volumes of encyclopaedias or even telephone books, but it makes a lot of sense anyway to invest in a set of short dumb- bells.

Depending on your training objective, you should choose between short dumb-bells with exchangeable discs (precise and quick to adjust) or gym dumb-bells (can be used in a wide range due to foot loops, low weight, starting at 2 lbs – even can be used for endurance sports, for example when jogging or walking).

*Training focus:* Strengthening (shoulders, arms, chest)
*Price:* Starting at about £ 12 UK/$ 20 US/$ 27 Cdn up

**Weight Cuffs**
Similar to the gym dumb-bells you can turn a simple gymnastic exercise like doing jumping jacks into a sweat producing, intensive, strengthening exercise. At the same time the weight cuffs have the advantage, that when fixing them onto the hand or foot joints, the range of movement will not be limited, the hands are free.
*Training focus:* Strengthening (extremities: arms, legs)
*Price:* Starting at £ 7 UK/$ 3,50 US/$ 17 Cdn up, weight starting at 1,5 kg

**AB-trainer or Sit-up Roller**
The frame is similar to the overroll bar which supports the curling-up movement and with its strengths the belly muscles without hurting the spine. When buying it you should pick one which is adjustable and has a safeguard so it will not slide around.
*Training focus:* Strengthening (abdominals)
*Price:* Starting at about £ 30 UK/$ 47 US/$ 70 Cdn up

**Bicycle Ergometer**
It does use up a little space in the living-room but is a great alternative – especially when the weather is bad – to keep your endurance and improve it. When buying one you should watch for an eddy-current brake and that the weight of the flywheel is around 15-20 kg. You will only have fun exercising if the step is round. Almost all bikes which meet these conditions come with a pulse reader and deliver the "tourdates" via display. These are usually not comparable to "outdoor-tours" – usually they are a little "flattering". Increasingly stepper and treads to use at home are offered – but tread-mills priced below £ 300 UK/$ 480 US/$ 690 Cdn up are not recommended you have to make a lot of compromises regarding the running pace and shock absorption.
*Training focus:* Endurance
*Price:* Starting at £ 200 UK/$ 330 US/$ 480 Cdn up (if the mentioned requirements are met)

**Gymnastic Mat**
Certainly a towel or a thick carpet are sufficient without getting pressure sores when lying down. More practical for endurance and strengthening gymnastics on the floor however is a gymnastic mat.
*Training focus:* Strengthening and endurance gymnastics
*Price:* Starting at about £ 15 UK/$ 25 US/$ 35 Cdn up.

**Home Fitness Centre**
This multi-function machine uses up a lot of space and since it is not really a decoration for the living-room, you need a good-sized hobby room. As a lot of compromises are made when trying to combine as many exercise varieties as possible, it will never even get close to those in commercial fitness centres. The strength lapse during certain exercises – in specific machines regulated by eccentric discs – is adverse. Furthermore a favourable orthopaedic, or even uncomfortable position, is often taken when doing the exercises. Cheap machines often are not really solid and because of this can make their use difficult or strongly restrict it.

*Training focus:* Strengthening/build-of up muscles
*Price:* Starting at about £ 200 UK/$ 330 US/$ 480 Cdn up (adjustable multi-function bench with weights/dumb-bells)

When using a combination of Therapeutic Band and skipping rope for example one has an alternative to the fitness centre which is only the size of a pack of cigarettes and can be used very well and diversified to train endurance, strength and co-ordination for a price of less than £ 6 UK/$ 10 US/$ 15 Cdn up.

**Be careful when seeing advertisements** which make great promises! There is no way to get the top-figure by only exercising ten minutes a day, regardless of what the producers of the equipment promise.

That is why you should very critically check the offer if it is promising spectacular things. "Wondermachines" often turn out to be duds. Often these advertisements and videos are made by irresponsible people who want to earn their money with the help of human vanity rather than the exercise equipment. Who will admit that he has not reached the training goal? That the goal could not have been reached with this equipment in the suggested time anyway is another story altogether.

## 3.4 The Right Choice – How to Find My Fitness Studio

If you intend to work-out in a fitness centre, you should first varify some details and compare how much you have to pay and what you get for it.

The best way to do this is to schedule a test-training which should be free of charge. Enclosed are the most important aspects you should take into consideration when chosing a studio and which you should check-out during the test training

### 1. Location

What was your first impression? Are the rooms spacious, light and aired well? Pay attention to cleanlinies and hygiene, especially in the changing-rooms and the ablutions section. Is the arrangement of the rooms well thought-out and easy to overlook? Is the equipment functional (a springy, shock- and sound-absorbing "swing" floor in the aerobic room) are there areas for gymnastic and stretching exercises (with mats)?

May children be brought along? Is there a "kiddie-corner" where they are being looked after?

What are your other main concerns? Do you attach great importance to what and how much is being offered in the relaxing-section. In many centres a sauna, Turkish bath, swimming-pool and fresh-air regions are a norm.

### 2. Consultation/Care

Ask about the qualification of coaches. Are qualified coaches (certified physical training instructors, physiotherapists etc) available not only during the test training but are they also available to talk to and to control the performance of exercises – especially for beginners? Are the trainers and reception-desk staff friendly and helpful? Is an individual training plan being made just for you? A fitness test or check is as recommended as the control and documentation of the training progress.

### 3. Equipment

You know your training objectives – is the equipment needed to get there available and in a sufficient number? Tight spots often develop on the ad-ductor and abductor machines, especially during rush-hour in the evening between 7 and 9 p.m. How good is the user comfort? Are the machines adjustable to your body size without a problem? Is the change of weights to determine the resistance women-specific – meaning you can adjust in small steps? Is the equipment steady and secure i.e. panelling of the weightcolumns – of importance if you take a child along? Are the machines cleaned and maintained well or are there stains from sweat residue visible on the padding? Many women like to use heart and circulation equipment like steppers, exercise bikes, tread-mills etc, often and intensively.

There should be plenty available because the average time of use for this apparatus is about 1/2 hour. Endurance equipment should be equipped with a heart rate monitor (at the handle bars) or with a Polar belt. The earclip often is not precise enough or out of order. The latest models have motivating programmes in their display like simulation of hills, pursuit races etc which are supposed to make the time fly by and increase the fun during the exercise.

### 4. Atmosphere/Ambiance
What do the other members look like? Are you comfortable around these people? You should pay special attention to these points: average age, ratio of men to women, dominating outfit, background music.

### 5. Further Things which could be of Interest for You
Parking places, bistro, massage, solarium, courses (aerobics, back and spine gymnastics, stretching, functional gymnastics and others). Is the ablutions section separated by gender or are days for women only offered.

### 6. Contracts
When signing a contract especially watch for clauses about the time it is valid for, automatic extensions (no more than three months) and periods of cancellation (maximum six weeks). If you want to make sure not to miss a period of cancellation, have a clause added before you sign it that the membership automatically ends at the end of the given time. There should be a special right to terminate the contract in case you move away, get pregnant or if there is a longer illness.

Overall you should feel comfortable. Many women prefer training in a studio for women only, which especially meets their demands and wishes.

## 3.5 Information on Courses Offered at Fitness Centres

A constantly increasing selection of courses being offered with new names and new ways to exercise – who can keep up with that? Callanetics – the hit in the fitness centres just recently – is already (for good reasons) mega out now!

### Aerobic – Low Impact
An exercise where one moves to music but one leg always stays on the ground (no jumps). Therefore it does not put too much strain on the joints.
*Training objective:* Co-ordination, endurance
*Target group:* Beginners, suitable for overweight people
*Remark:* If there is a variety of courses pay attention to a possible difficulty level.

### Aerobic – High Impact
In comparison to low impact aerobics tougher exercises (jump variations) for the heart circulation system as well as for the joints.
*Training objective:* Co-ordination, endurance
*Target group:* Advanced
*Remark:* Be careful of how much load you can handle (control of the pulse).

### Step Aerobic
By using "steps" as a kind of level where "height" can be adjusted, a well-proportioned programme can be offered, the work-out is mainly for the legs and the buttock.
*Training objective:* Co-ordination, strength endurance
*Target group:* Everybody because it can be adjusted to anybody's level.

 ### Slide
This used to be the summer training for ice skaters, now it is a good way to get the circulation going and to work on the upper thighs.
*Training objective:* Co-ordination, strength endurance training
*Target group:* No limits.
*Remark:* The sliding to the side on a sliding mat is good for the joints and similar to the movement when iceskating or rollerblading.

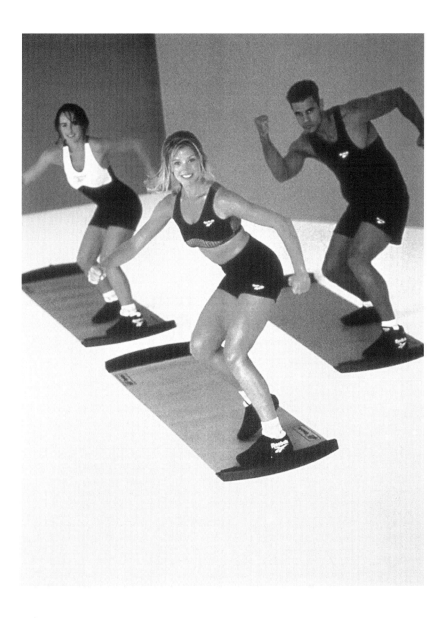

*Figure 8: Easy on the joints and very efficient – sliding*

### Fatburner

A good exercise to get the fat metabolism going.

*Training objective:* Endurance, weight reduction

*Target group:* Beginners, overweight people

### Bodyshaping/Bodyforming/Bodytoning

Programmes for the whole body to improve your figure by tightening the muscles.

*Training objective:* Strengthening, improvement of the figure

*Target group:* No limits

### Hip-Hop/Funk/Cardio Jazz

Working out to the sound of different styles of music; a mix between aerobic and dance components. In comparison with aerobic the choreography is more demanding.

*Training objective:* Endurance, co-ordination, flexibility

*Target group:* Preferably for people with advanced training

### Spinal Gymnastics

Programme to work-out the trunk musculature. In particular muscular imbalances are supposed to be "repaired" by bending/stretching and strengthening exercises.

*Training objective:* Strength, flexibility

*Target group:* Recommended for people with minor back problems e.g. for people who work at a desk.

*Remark:* Doing spinal gymnastics is not a therapy but rather a precaution. If you suffer from major back problems, especially in the intervertebral disc area, you should consult a physician.

# 4 Nutrition

## 4.1 The Ideal Diet during Sporting Activity

People who are consciously active should eat sensibly to reach their training objectives and to increase performance. We eat food that is too fat, too sweet and too much. This, combined with a lack of movement, stress and other negative environmental influences, does not only lead to problems with the body but creates health problems as well.

There are far too many so called "empty calories" on our menu: sweets, sodas, cake, white bread, alcohol, meats and sausages which are high in fat. Because of this we eat incorrectly as well as too much. The results: deposits of fat, being overweight and a reduction of one's performance ability.

In order to maintain the human organism, three basic nutriments are necessary:
• carbohydrates (quickly supply energy)
• fats (supply energy and store it)
• and protein (building-material).
In addition to that, vitamines, minerals, trace elements and water play an important role for metabolism.

| Nutriment | in reality | ideal |
|---|---|---|
| fat | 38% | 30% |
| protein | 12% | 12% |
| complex carbohydrates | 24% | 48% |
| (high quality starch) | | |
| simple carbohydrates | 18% | 10% |
| (food and beverages containing sugar) | | |
| alcohol | 8% | 0% |

Figure 9: Nutrition actual and target figures (according to HAMM 1990)

Without getting to deep into the topic of nutrition, which is covered very detailed in special literature we would like to offer some basic advice:

1. Use nutritional density instead of empty calories. Carbohydrates do not make you fat but fit. Therefore you should increase the complex carbo-hydrate part in your diet. Best-suited for this in main dishes are whole-meal pasta, high quality rice and potatoes. More than just a positive side effect, when increasing the intake of fibre your digestion will also improve.

2. Reduce the fats in your nutrition. However there is no doubt that the human body has a basic need for fat. These essential (indispensable) fats which are absolutely necessary for the organism (fat acids) are mostly found in vegetable oils.
   Especially avoid lunch meats/sandwich fillings with lots of fat, sausages which are high in fat, fat gravy etc. Rather pick poultry and fish when chosing. "Fat dips" are also unwise as are desserts, cakes, chocolate, whole milk, cheese (watch for the percentage of fat in it!), potato chips, nuts and olives.

3. Cover your demand for protein mainly with vegetable proteins (i.e. tofu) as well as with milk products which are low in fat. Because of a high percentage of fat, cholesterol and uric acid meat should be on your menu very seldom.

4. Put an emphasis on food which contains a lot of water such as lettuce, cucumbers, (water-) melons etc. These contain vitamins, minerals, fibre and are low in fat and calories.
   The same goes for fresh fruit. The high proportion of enzymes in a lot of fruit (pineapples, papayas) speeds up the digestive system. Since fruit juices have a lot of calories they should be watered down with mineral water.

5. Get away from the traditional eating habits! A lot of small meals, spread out over the course of the day are better than three big ones.

6. Be cautious when using sugar, salt or alcohol.

7. Not only eating habits but also drinking habits must be right. Most athletes (male as well as female) drink too little, at the wrong time and mostly the wrong beverages as well.
Do not wait until your are thirsty to drink when you are doing sport because by that time the performance as well as the concentration level will be down; drink at regular periods. Usually you should drink 2-3 litres of liquids such as mineral water, herbal teas or juices, thinned down with water each day. You should be careful not to use up a high amount of your daily calorie demand with the beverages. While doing sport activities, the body can lose up to 1,5 litres of liquid in one hour. Naturally this loss has to be replaced as soon as possible after the perspiration producing activities.
Specific electrolytic beverages are ideal after sport, but they are expensive. A watered-down apple juice to which a magnesium mixture can be added to if an intensive endurance training has been undertaken will get the same results.

8. Your diet plan should not consist of too many "not advised" items. On the one hand everything prohibited has a big appeal to it, on the other hand the partaking of, and pleasure of good eating is not to be ignored when eating.

Basically your food, regardless of the goals you have set for yourself, should be filling, taste good, easy to prepare and not too expensive.

# 4.2 Nutritional Supplements

When you use healthy, diversified food, and taking into consideration the recommendations of the previous chapter, supplements to your diet will not be necessary.

If it is not possible to turn this into reality on a day-to-day basis however, you can prevent malnutrition by taking dietary supplements such as vitamin or mineral mixtures.

*Recommendation:* ACE & Selen, calcium and calium

When doing intensive endurance training, you should make sure to re-place the minerals which were lost with the sweat: magnesium, natrium and calcium should also be taken as a supplement. In autumn and winter a supplement of vitamin C helps the immune system.

In order to increase the mobility of fat acids, products with carnitin have been on the market for some time. Please note that carnitin alone cannot burn fat, only when doing intensive endurance training do you reach the results wished for. Yet the body mostly supplies itself with this substance by producing it itself. Taking carnitin for a long time bears the risk of the body reducing its production.

Glucose helps mostly during short-termed loading, for endurance or sport games it is rather unsuitable.

A number of remedies on the market, like Gelée Royale, Coenzym Q10 or energy drinks (Red Bull and others) bring positive effects to heart rate, en-durance capacity and regeneration time. Last but not least because of their price use of these products makes sense mostly for sports women who take part in competitions.

We do not want to get further into the subject of nutritional supplements since this market changes daily, so tomorrow's new "wonder pills" with "surprising effects" will be on offer.

# 4.3 Dieting and Fasting

Please forget the kind of diet coures which some magazines use to in-crease their meagre circulation. They only affect those diets which lack the nutrition needed, and will empty your wallet in the long run.

As mentioned before, dieting and fasting will bring short-term success when the calorie intake is significantly decreased. Yet often you can notice the "jo-jo-effect" which means that weight has been gained again shortly af-ter the diet. When fasting rigorously you often lose muscles in addition to water, meaning active body substance, which often gets replaced by fat when putting on weight again. An extremely negative effect.

Fat can be reduced only by muscles for even when resting a trained muscle uses up energy.

Furthermore doing sport and fasting does not go together. When dieting the body reduces itself to a pilot light, the absolute necessary only, the basic turnover goes down. Therefore get moving instead of fasting! Those who only diet lose less than those who participate in a combined diet and sports programme. In addition to that an active life prevents a fast weight gain after a diet.

There is no doubt that a carefully chosen diet helps to reach the goal of losing fat, showing first results in a short time and this definitely helps to improve motivation.

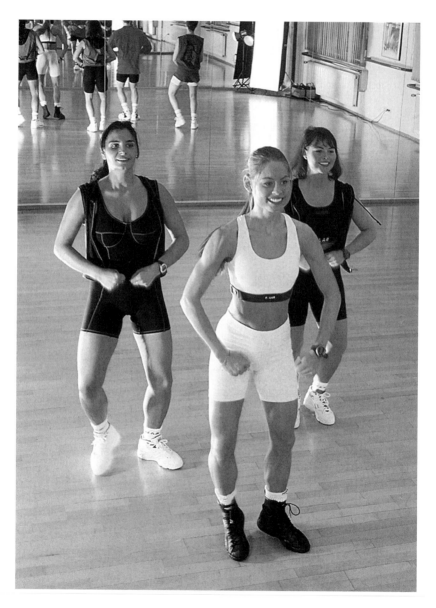

*Figure 10: Motivation: Working-out in a group*

# 5 Motivation

All over the world sports women talk about motivation. Especially in top sport it is realised that if performance capacity is about the same, in most cases the sports woman who is in the "healthier state of mind", that is the one who is motivated more, moves ahead. Coaches are celebrated as "artists of motivation" in the media; often psychologists are part of the coaching staff.

I admit that the aspect of a record performance is of no importance in this book or for your training schedule, but some "psychotricks" might be helpful for you too, to reach your objectives.

You have probably noticed yourself that your motivation is subject to seasonal inconsistencies, and that your mood swings have an effect on your activities. Also not all weathers promise fun when doing sport outside. There are lots of excuses as well as hindrances, important is the right strategy to get rid of them.

### 1. Setting one's Aims

Set yourself individual, clear objectives. The goal should be set realisticly, meaning it should be attainable and it should be adjusted to your present level of performance. But it is necessary for you to challenge yourself. By buying this book you have taken the important first step.

You have made the first decision about changing your life habits. To be more precise, ask yourself the questions (perhaps you should also write them down):

- What do I want to achieve?
- When do I want to reach this objective?
- How much time (daily/weekly) do I have – do I want to invest?

Work out personal "contracts" and do not forget to consider the reward.

Now concentrate on the chosen, positively defined objective until you have reached it.

Helpfull are objectives you can measure objectively and you can mark in stages (for example loss of weight). Yet more important than the success on the scales seems to be the success which cannot be measured in numbers, which is the enhancement of your well-being and your performance capacity.

## 2. Training Partners

An advice everybody will give you is to look for an appropriate training partner (male or female) or a group. Reciprocal incentive, appointments scheduled together (it is easier to cancel your own appointment than those made with others) and conversations in a group make it easier to get over lows when they occur occasionally. Yet there is always the risk of being challenged too much or not enough because of your partner. Furthermore, it will be difficult to reach your objective all by yourself once the partner has quit.

## 3. Training Times

Make yourself some concrete free time which will be reserved for training and sport activities only. It will be easier with a plan as simple as possible, for example Mondays, Wednesdays, Fridays at 6 p.m. – or a daily programme at a set time.

*Try not to make any compromises here – these times are yours for your sport.*

# II HOW YOU EXERCISE RIGHT

# 1 Fitness Test

In order to achieve a well thought out, promising training session this is what you should do:

**1. Set an objective:** As mentioned in the chapter "motivation" already, you should set yourself clear objectives.

**2. Determination of the "current performance level":** In order to determine the difference in your current status and your training objectives you need a diagnosis of your current fitness which you can obtain by doing some tests. For this purpose you should also write down your weight, abdominal girth and the percentage of fat in your body. Resting pulse and blood pressure are important measurements as well. To get some blood results and pulmonary function results you should consult a doctor. That way it is easier to measure the level of the cholesterol by regular endurance training.

**3. Training programme:** Combine suitable methods and ways to reach your objective.

**4. Control:** By performing these tests (if possible under the same circumstances, weekly or monthly) you can easily compare the results at the beginning with the one you want to reach.

## 1.1 Endurance

**Cooper test:** While controversial in competitive sports, the Cooper test has established itself in the fitness and health areas. It is easy to perform without a lot of remedies, and enables a fast, affirmative evaluation.

The only thing required for it is a – if possible – flat set measured-out round course (ideal would be the running track of a sports field) and a stopwatch. The distance you put behind you in twelve minutes will be measured and it will be decisive for your aerobic capacity. A pace should be set which allows you to breathe without problems; walking pauses are allowed.

| age-group judgement | 20-29 | 30-39 | 40-49 | 50-59 | 60-69 |
|---|---|---|---|---|---|
| outstanding | over 2320 | over 2220 | over 2140 | over 2080 | over 1980 |
| very good | 2160 2320 | 2080 2220 | 2000 2140 | 1900 2080 | 1760 1890 |
| good | 1970 2150 | 1900 2070 | 1790 1990 | 1700 1890 | 1580 1750 |
| medium | 1790 1960 | 1700 1890 | 1580 1780 | 1500 1690 | 1390 1570 |
| weak | 1540 1780 | 1500 1690 | 1410 1570 | 1340 1490 | 1250 1380 |
| very weak | under 1540 | under 1500 | under 1410 | under 1340 | under 1250 |

*Figure 11: Interpretation Cooper test (running distance after twelve minutes in metre/valuation. Valid for women only. Statements according to BÖS, 1996)*

# 1.2 Strength

Only strength endurance can be tested in fitness training. Maximum strength is not suitable to be measured. The test exercises should be easy and you should be able to perform them anywhere.

### a) Test exercise for the muscles of the abdomen
Held crunches propped up against the wall

**Execution:** Lift the upper body until your elbows touch the upper thighs (start of the timing). Try to stay in this position as long as possible without forcing your breathing.

#### Valuation

| | |
|---|---|
| under 15 s | bad |
| 16-30 s | moderate |
| 31-45 s | medium |
| 46-60 s | good |
| over 60 s | very good |

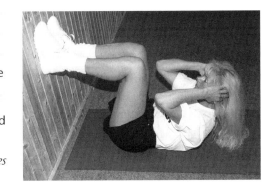

*Figure 12: Testing the muscles of the abdomen*

### b) Test exercise for the hip and leg muscles
Lower arm supports backwards

**Execution:** Lift up the body, your weight rests on your elbows and heels. Stay in this position as long as possible without forcing your breathing.

#### Valuation

| | |
|---|---|
| under 15 s | bad |
| 16-30 s | moderate |
| 31-45 s | medium |
| 46-60 s | good |
| over 60 s | very good |

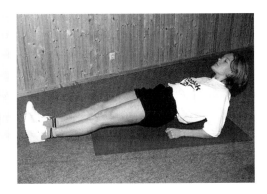

*Figure 13: Test hip and leg muscles*

### c) Exercise to test the chest, shoulder, arm musculature
Knee push-ups

**Execution:** Lying on your belly, you place your palms next to your shoulders. The lower thighs are angled upwards, the feet are crossed over each other. Now you take turns stretching and bending your arms.
*Important:* Tension on the shoulder blade and stabilisation of the lumbar vertebrae. When going down inhale, when pushing up exhale.

**Valuation**

| | |
|---|---|
| 0-5 reps | bad |
| 6-10 reps | moderate |
| 11-14 reps | medium |
| 15-18 reps | good |
| over 18 reps | very good |

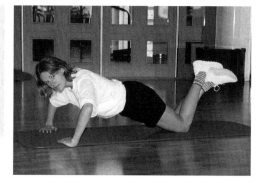

*Figure 14: Test knee push-ups*

### d) Exercise to test the musculature of the thighs
Squatting against a wall

**Execution:** Your back is pressed against the wall. Lower thigh to upper thigh and upper thigh to trunk are each in a 90° angle. Hold this position as long as possible while continuing to breath calmly.

**Valuation**

| | |
|---|---|
| 0-30 s | bad |
| 31-60 s | moderate |
| 61-90 s | medium |
| 91-120 s | good |
| 120 s and more | very good |

*Figure 15: Test upper thigh musculature*

# 1.3 Flexibility

*a) Exercise to test the flexibility of the trunk/back of the leg*
(not suitable for people with back problems)

**Execution:** Sit in front of a wall in a way that when you straighten your knees, the soles of your feet push against the wall. Now move your hands towards the wall while keeping your back straight. Make sure that your motion is very slow. After a few carefull "warm-ups" try to stay in the position you can reach for a maximum for two seconds.

## Valuation

Fingertips are farther than 10 cm away from the wall     bad
0-10 cm distance from the wall     moderate
Touching the wall with both middle fingers     medium/good
Touching the wall with both thumbs     very good

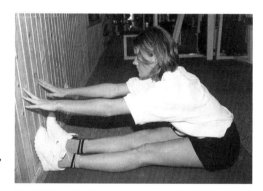

*Figure 16: Test flexibility of the trunk*

*b) Exercise to test the chest/shoulder area*
A general statement can be made referring to the flexibility in this area by only slightly changing the position of your arms during exercise 1.2 d (squatting against a wall). You should be able to push against the wall with both lower arms.

More specific results about the flexibility in the shoulder girth can be given when doing the test "dislocation of the shoulders"

**Execution:** A stick is being pulled over the head behind the back - the arms are stretched out. Systematically shorten the width of the grip until you can barely pull the stick behind you without bending your arms.
   You measure the smallest width of the grip and the width of your shoulder.
   *Measurement:* width of the grip-shoulder width

**Valuation:**

| | |
|---|---|
| over 73 cm | bad |
| 62-72 cm | moderate |
| 55-61 cm | medium |
| 47-54 cm | good |
| less than 46 cm | very good |

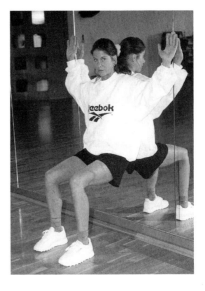

*Figure 17: Flexibility test for the chest/shoulder region*

# 2 Exercises

## 2.1 Endurance

**Which forms of sport are suitable for an optimum endurance training?**
Recommended are those with a minimum possibility of damaging the body and which lead to a maximum of positive health results for the heart circulation system.

**Running** in the form of a long-distance race on a flat ground is very suitable. In a well-proportioned long-distance run the lowest build-up of lactate in comparison to the oxygen intake can be noticed. Compared to the amount of oxygen inhaled, the increase in blood pressure is insignificant. There are no complicated technical preconditions necessary when running. There are no costs except for adequate running shoes. Running is not bound to a certain area or time. Problems only occur if people are very obese or have damaged joints.

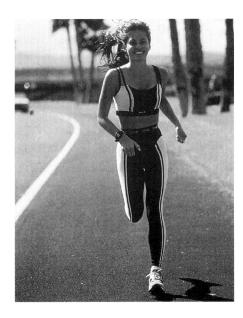

*Figure 18: The correct loading while running due to POLAR measurement of the heart rate.*

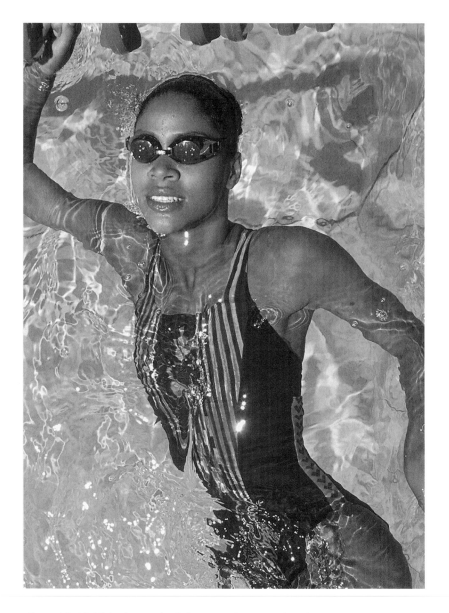

*Figure 19: Multiple demands of the musculature: swimming*

*osteoarthritis*

**Cycling** is a good alternative to running, expecially when being over-weight or suffering from degenerative joint diseases (arthrosis). Likewise, the ratio of oxygen intake and the increase of pressure and lactate produc-tion is low. The local use of strength is higher as it is when running. If the upper thigh musculature is not trained this often puts a limit to the perfor-mance and heart rates of training standard will hardly be attained. Be-cause of the greater local muscle tension in the upper thigh when step-ping on the pedals the blood pressure goes up a little more compared to running. In order to prevent getting fatigue quickly, a lower gear should be used, meaning you should cycle in a high-stepping frequency with a low stepping resistance.

**Run and bike** is a lively combination between cycling and jogging. Usual-ly two people start with one bike – one person jogs, the partner cycles next to him/her. After a pre-arranged time (between one and four min-utes), or distance, you take turns. The changing exercise intensity especial-ly stimulates the adjustability of the heart circulation system. The constant change makes training more lively. It is an ideal possibility for couples who have different performance capacities, to work-out together without one of them being over or understrained, because the running speed al-ways sets the pace. You can also adjust a difference in capacity by using different running distances.

When **swimming**, many muscles are being used and it is a sport which overweight or handicapped people can participate in too. But often swim-ming turns into bathing, and looking at it from an endurance training point of view, most people can do this only with breast stroke. This is not without problems for the knees and the lumbar vertebrae spine – to swim the crawl or on your back (in public pools not always recommended) would be better. To measure your pulse in the water, we have the follow-ing orientation help: 160 - your age.

**Rollerblading** is a big trend right now. Certainly sport trends should be looked at thoroughly but rollerblading seems to establish itself in all age-groups – for good reasons! The equipment, once used by ice hockey pro-fessionals during summer training, now offers joint-protecting endurance, fun, and, contrary to cycling or jogging, the inside as well as the outside of the thighs are used, too. A complete set of protection gear (helmet, wrist, knee and elbow protection) is very necessary and the learning of a of good braking technique. It is best to take part in a course for this and find flat stretches with no traffic when first practicing.

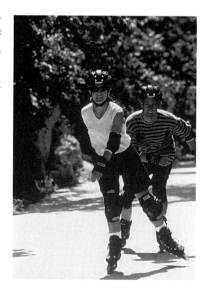

*Figure 20: Trendy and healthy: Rollerblading – if technique and equipment are right*

Often you read about the idea that cardiovascular training can be performed by a muscle training with low intensities and no pauses. This might be correct for strength endurance training but is totally different when looking closer at the activity of the heart when under load.

If the muscle is overloaded with 15% over its normal capacity, the pressure of the muscle, on the vessels and the blood flow decreases. When greater than 50% of the maximum strength this compression leads to a total stop of circulation. When running, the vessel, of the body widen so the heart will not be burdened in addition to the volume work because it pumps more blood with increased pressure as well. But this is exactly what happens during strength training. The blood pressure goes up considerably even when only small muscle groups are being used.

The heart muscle follows the same regularities as the other muscles. When being inactive, its performance capacity goes down, when training regularly, it increases.

The heart muscle responds to work loads which occur for example when running a long distance with physiological hyperthropy, meaning a harmonic growth of all parts of the heart. Due to its volume of work the hollow area increases, because more blood per heart beat can be pumped into the periphery. This is the precondition for an economical heart rate when resting and during submaximum strains, because the heart does not have to beat as often for the same amount of blood. The motor of the heart will not have to be powered up as much.

Due to these considerations we can observe:
Strength training is an excellent way to compensate muscular deficits, inbalances and – as a result of this – posture and capacity problems and to get many more already mentioned positive effects on an orthopedical as well as an internist's level. For optimum heart circulation training however, we have to use forms like running and biking.

## 2.2 Warm-up

In order to tolerate loads from the beginning as well as to be protected against injuries, the body has to be set in an increased capacity stand-by. This is suppose to get an increased reaction readiness of the central nervous system, a higher muscle temperature, and a more intensive metabolism. The increase of the heart- and breathing volume per minute provides a better recycling of metabolic dross and carbon dioxide.

The increased reaction readiness of the central nervous system improves the co-ordination during the individual exercises and prevents injuries. Due to the higher muscle temperature the frictional resistance in the muscles is lowered and this results in more elasticity and a higher contraction speed. When the body temperature rises the cartilage tissue of the sections lying on top of each other within the joints get thicker. This improves the distribution of pressure and enables the joints to take more load.

These points confirm how important a right warm-up is before the workout. Summing it all up you can say: A warmed-up muscle has a bigger capacity and is not as likely to get injured.

You can do a warm-up by rowing, climbing stairs, cycling, jogging, jumping on one spot or on a trampoline. Skipping ropes might be too exhausting for the beginner, and the heart rate will go up too much. Mostly in fitness-centres you will find bicycle ergometers, steppers and or running belts in the "cardio-area".

In order to get the effect mentioned, the warm-up time should take about 10-15 minutes. The optimum heart rate, depending on age and shape – should be at about 120 beats per minute.

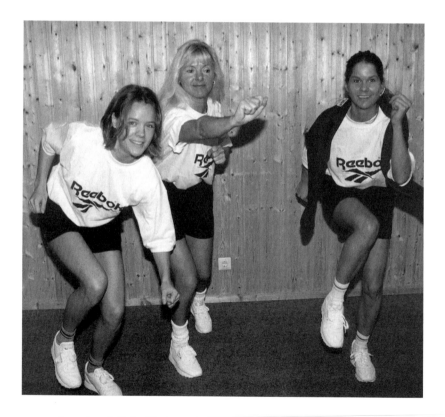

*Figure 21: Jumping to the side (A2)/Running while shadow-boxing (A3)/ Diagonal knee and elbow (A4)*

# 2.3 Stretching

Muscles, tendons and ligaments are flexible structures. They can get stiff, and due to this the range of movement will be restricted.

Intensive, sometimes unilateral muscle training and one-sided routine loads which occur during the day-to-day work lead to a shortening of the muscle if you do not counteract this by stretching. But how do you stretch correctly?

Excessive bouncing, absorbing the shock, swinging etc meaning common "stretching techniques" bear the danger that through stretching reflexes proprioceptive tensions will build up, the joints will not be balanced out all the way and this will allow compensation movements in the adjoining joints. In the muscles are so called muscle spindles which control the tension and length status of the muscles through the reflex system and protect it from injuries.

If a sudden and strong stretching of the muscles occurs, as usually is the case when bouncing or absorbing the shock, the muscle spindle sends a signal which will cause the contraction of the muscle. The muscle consequently contracts itself to avoid being ruptured.

Instead of a stretching, the opposite happens. There is nothing amiss about a light, controlled bouncing in the final position of a stretching exercise however. Very unphysiological to improve the flexibility are rotation movements of body parts which by nature are not meant to be used for this: circling of the head, trunk, etc.

One of the most commonly used stretching technics is the CHRS- method (contract, hold, relax, stretch). This means that each stretching exercise will be broken down in three phases: a strong static tension (8-10 s) followed by a short relaxing phase (2-3 s). This reduces the muscular reflecting resistance considerably against the stretching, the muscle can now be stretched best (15-20 s).

Here is a stretching programme for the whole body with the eleven most important exercises:

## Stretching Exercise S5: Back of Thighs

**Contraction:** The stretched leg presses strongly into the mat with the heel. Stay in this position for 8-10 s while breathing calmly.

**Relaxing::** 2-3 s

**Stretching:** Push the upper body over the stretched leg; the spine remains straight. Keep the feeling of tension on the back of the upper thigh for 15-20 s. The point of the foot should be pulled upwards.

**Possible faults:** Round back, moving your pelvis sideways, the knee not being stretched

**Hint:**
If you have knee problems make sure you have an adequate support.

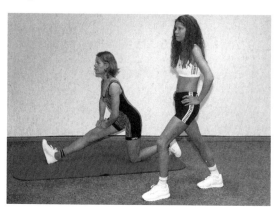

*Figure 22:*
*Stretching exercise S5:*
*Back of upper thigh (left)*
*Stretching exercise S6:*
*Calf (right)*

## Stretching Exercise S6: Calf

**Contraction:** Point your toes upwards.

**Relaxing!**

**Stretching:** Starting from a "step" position the center of gravity will be pushed over the front leg. Hereby you must pay attention that the back leg is stretched; the heel of the leg in the back has to stay on the ground.

**Possible faults:** The feet are not pointing forwards.

**Hint:** If you often wear shoes with a heel (often leads to a shortening of the calf musculature) you should especially pay attention to this exercise.

## Stretching Exercise S7: Abductor Muscles

**Contraction:**       The knee of the leg which is angled crossways presses upwards against the resistance of the hand.

**Relaxing!**
**Stretching:**        The hand presses the knee onto the ground, the trunk rests opposite

**Possible faults:**   Shoulder blade of the stretched sidelifts the ground

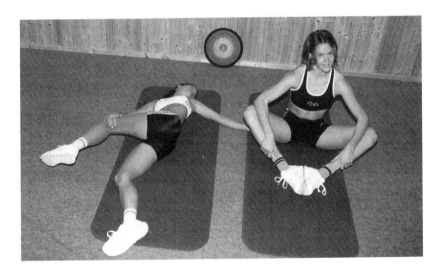

*Figure 23:   Stretching exercise S7: Abductor muscles (left); S8: Abductor muscles (right)* Stretching

## Exercise S8: Adductor Muscles

**Contraction:**       While sitting, the legs are slightly opened and angled and press against the resistance of the lower arm.

**Relaxing!**
**Stretching:**        The arms are pushing the legs downwards

**Possible faults:**   Round back

**Hint:**              This exercise mainly stretches the short adductor muscles which tend to shorten.

## Stretching Exercise S9: Front of the Thigh/Hip Flexor

**Contraction:**      Lying on the side, you bend your upper leg
                      backwards. The foot is pressing against the hand.
**Relaxing!**
**Stretching:**       The hand pulls the foot backwards and up, at the
                      same time you push your hip forwards.
**Possible faults:**  Evasive movement of the lower thigh, knees not
                      close

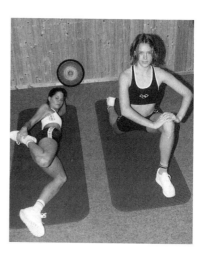

*Figure 24:*
*Stretching exercise S9: Front of the*
*upper thigh/bending the hip (left)*
*Stretching exercise S10: Bending the*
*hip/front of the upper thigh (right)*

## Stretching Exercise S10: Hip Flexor/Front of the Thigh

**Contraction:**      Wide split step. Press the foot of the leg positioned
                      in the back "into the ground".
**Relaxing!**
**Stretching:**       Stay in this split step position and try to push the
                      pelvis down in the direction of the front heel. The
                      upper body remains upright.
**Possible faults:**  The front thigh is not vertical.
**Hint:**             The hip flexor is one of the muscles which tends to be
                      shortened. It is also very difficult to
                      stretch. Only an intensive stretching on a regular
                      basis improves the flexibility.

## Stretching Exercise S11: Lower Back

Not suitable for people who have problems with the intervertebral discs

| | |
|---|---|
| **Contraction:** | Lying on your belly lift your upper body a little. |
| **Relaxing!** | |
| **Stretching:** | While standing, you bend forward the upper body, drop to your knees and grip around the knees with both arms. Now try to slowly straighten up your knees as much as possible. |
| **Hint:** | Ideal preparation prior to training of the abdominal muscles because of the resisting effect of the flexed un-stretched back muscles. |

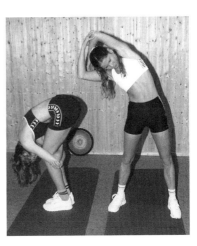

*Figure 25:*
*Stretching exercise S11: Lower back (left)*
*Stretching exercise S12: Trunk side/triceps*
*(right)*

## Stretching Exercise S12: Trunk Side/Triceps

| | |
|---|---|
| **Contraction:** | While standing, put your arm in an angle behind your head, the hand between the shoulder blades. The elbow presses in the opposite hand. |
| **Relaxing!** | |
| **Stretching:** | Pull the arm behind the head. Bend your trunk along to the side in the direction being pulled. |
| **Possible faults:** | Swerving of the trunk. |

## Stretching Exercise S13: Chest/Shoulder Exercises

**Contraction:**     The hand of the arm which is stretched out to the side presses onto the mat.

**Relaxing!**

**Stretching:**     Head and upper body are turned to the side and up with the help of the propped up arm.

**Possible faults:**     The shoulder which is to be stretched is not on the ground, the stretched-out arm is not bent in an angle.

**Alternative:**     This exercise can also be performed while standing at a doorframe or at a column.

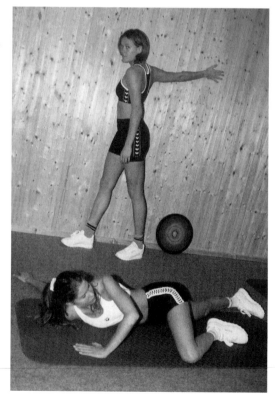

*Figure 26:*
*Stretching exercise S13:*
*Chest/shoulder recumbent –*
*alternative standing*

## Stretching Exercise S14: Back of the Neck/Cervix Region

**Contraction:** While standing, fold your hands behind your head, the back of the head presses against the palms.

**Relaxing!**
**Stretching:** The folded hands pull the head forward and down – the chin in the direction of the breastbone.

**Hint:**
Due to the sensitive structure of the cervical vertebra area the head may only be pulled forward and down very carefully and slowly.

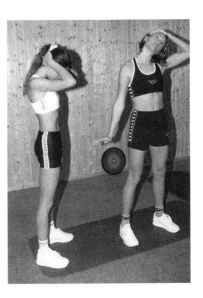

*Figure 27:*
*Stretching exercise S14: Back of the neck/cervix region (left); Stretching exercise S15: Side of the neck (right)*

## Stretching Exercise S15: Side of the Neck

**Contraction:** The hand reaches for the temple, the head presses sideways against the hand.

**Relaxing!**
**Stretching:** The other hand grips over the head and softly pulls the head to the side.

**Possible faults:** Pulling too strongly

**Hint:** While stretching consciously push the free arm downwards.

Exercises 9 and 10 are ideal for small stretching breaks at the desk.

## 2.4 Gymnastics

### a) Musculature of the Trunk

*Remark:* Abdominal and back muscles are postural muscles and should be exercised slowly. Therefore you should not insist on a certain repetition number. By doing so you often call for a too fast execution of the exercise. To aim for a certain time is more sensible.

### Exercise G16: Crunches (Abdominal, straight)

**Execution:** While lying on your back you bend your legs so the thigh forms a right angle to the hip and the lower leg forms a right angle to the upper leg.

The feet may be propped against a wall or simply be held up in the air. You can also prop up your lower legs on a work-out bench, or a chair, if the right angle can still be obtained.

From this position, depending on your performance capacity, you lift your head and shoulder girdle – the line of sight is diagonally forward. By holding up the legs the delicate lumbar vertebrae region remains protected on the ground. Stay at the highest point for a short time and then slowly move back to the initial position without putting your head on the ground.

**Remark:** The correct position of the arms is discussed controversial. They can be moved forward passing the upper thighs (the hands are pushing against an imaginary resistance), or can be crossed in front of the chest. Previous experience shows that a lot of women have problems crossing their head in this position due to their weak neck muscles. Here it is helpful to cross the hands behind the head in order to support it. But the elbows have to point outwards then.

**Possible faults:** The hands folded behind the back will be used to get going.

**Variation:** To make the exercise more difficult, the hands may be folded behind the neck.

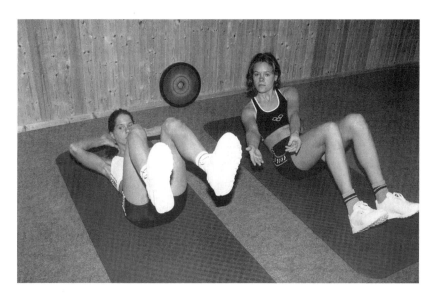

*Figure 28:*
*Exercise G16: Crunches (straight abdominals) (left); Exercise G17: Diagonal*
*crunches (diagonal abdominals) (right)*

## *Exercise G17: Diagonal Crunches (diagonal abdominals)*

**Execution:**    While lying on your back with propped up feet (heels strongly pushed into the support), both hands will be moved forward, passing the hip alternately left and right of it.

**Variation:**    Move the right elbow toward the left knee and vice versa. Stretch and bend your legs accordingly.

## Exercise G18: Pressing the Knee
### (static loading/diagonal abdominals)

**Execution:** Lying on the back, the left arm presses against the bent knee. Switch after 15-20 s. A static but gentle exercise.

**Remark:** Pay attention to a steady breathing.

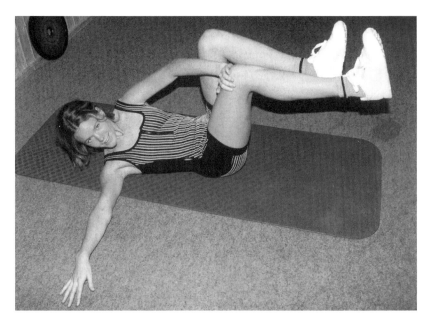

*Figure 29: Exercise G18: Pressing the knee (static loading/stomach diagonal)*

## Exercise G19: Lifting the Leg while Lying on the Side (trunk side)

**Execution:** While lying on the side, the stretched out legs should be lifted together and lowered again; without the lower foot touching the ground.

**Possible faults:** Pelvis falls backwards or forwards

**Varieties:** a) The exercise is easier if the legs are angled.
b) The upper leg lifted up a little more from the final position.

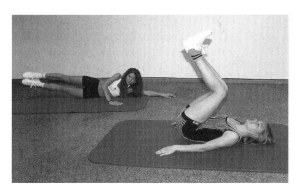

*Figure 30:*
*Exercise G19: Lifting the leg out of a side position (trunk side) (left)*
*Exercise G20: Lifting the pelvis (straight abdominal musculature) (right)*

## Exercise G20: Lifting up the Pelvis (straight abdominal musculature)

**Execution:** While lying on the back, the hip and knee joints are bent right-angled. Now the knees are moved slowly towards the shoulder, the pelvic bone remains lifted up a little.

**Possible faults:** A too fast execution of the exercise. Lifting the lumbar spine, forcing one's breath.

**Varieties:** From a lying position the angled legs are moved backwards until the buttock does not touch the ground anymore. The smaller the angle between hip and upper thigh, the easier the exercise. The exercise is started by a strong contraction of the stomach muscles, pressure of the lumbar vertebrae onto the support mat and slight tilting of the pelvis bones towards the ribs.

## Exercise G21: Diagonal Lifting of the Arm and the Leg (back/shoulder/buttock)

**Execution:** Lying on the belly (arms extended forwards), you alternately pick up the opposite extremities (left arm – right leg and vice versa). While doing this you have to build up a good body posture by actively pressing the tips of the feet into the support mat and flexing the upper thigh, buttock and stomach muscles. You look down onto the ground, the point of your nose almost touching it.

**Possible faults:** Missing body tension, knees on the ground, head in the neck

**Remarks:** If there are problems with abdominal tension or hollow back you should prop a pillow or something similar under your belly or pull one leg forward sideways (by doing that you can not slide to the side during the work-out anymore).

*Figure 31:*
*Exercise G21: Diagonal arm leg lifting (left)*
*Exercise G22: Alternately lifting shoulder and leg (right)*

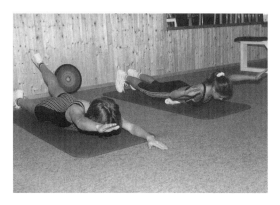

## Exercise G22: Alternately Lifting Shoulder/Leg

**Execution:** Lying on your stomach (arms are pulled forward in a u-formed angled) at first you lift the shoulder girdle and the arms off the ground. Stay this way for a moment and then lower them again. Now lift your legs in a way that the upper thighs will have as little contact as possible to the ground. Perform alternately.

**Possible faults:** Forcing one's breath, head in the neck

## Exercise G23: Lifting the Pelvis (back, buttock, back of thighs)

**Execution:** While lying on your back the legs are angled and the feet put onto the ground. Head and shoulders stay on the ground while the pelvis is lifted up until the body is stretched and a straight line is built from the knees up to the shoulders. If you are not used to this exercise, the arms can stay on the ground as a support, otherwise they will also be lifted up – the inner sides of the hands point up upwards.

**Varieties:** a) Dynamic performance: Take turns lifting and lowering the pelvis (no contact with the ground) b) To increase the exercise you can take turns stretching one leg so the described straight line goes all the way to the heel. If there is a lack of stabilisation, the pelvis can lower itself on the side of the extended leg.

**Possible faults:** Tipping the pelvis to one side

*Figure 32:Exercise G23: Lifting up the pelvis (back, buttock, back of thighs) (left)*

*Exercise G24: Picking up the trunk with the help of the knee (back extensor, buttock) (right)*

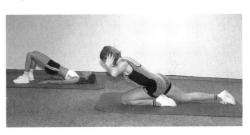

## Exercise G24: Picking up the Trunk with the Help of the Knee (back extensor, buttock)

**Execution:** From a bench position one leg will be pulled under the trunk, the other remains extended almost all the way. The hands rest on the forehead or the temples, not in the neck. Slowly lift your trunk until your back is extended. Do not lower the arms in between the repetitions. When getting exhausted, switch to the other knee.

**Possible faults:** Perform the movement too intensive, head tipped or overextended.

## Exercise G25: Leg lift in Lower Arms push up Position
### (whole body stabilisation/strengthening)

**Execution:** Propped up on knees, balls of the feet and elbows, the knees will be lifted up 5-10 cm while the back stays straight. The bigger the chosen angle between the trunk and thigh the more strenuous and difficult it will be to keep the back stabilised. Therefore this provides a good possibility when there are performance differences within training groups.

**Possible faults:** Moving the buttock upwards. The lumbar spine is not extended.

**Varieties:** Advanced sports people can additionally lift one foot to increase intensity of the exercise. When doing so you should pay attention to the hip region – it should stay straight.

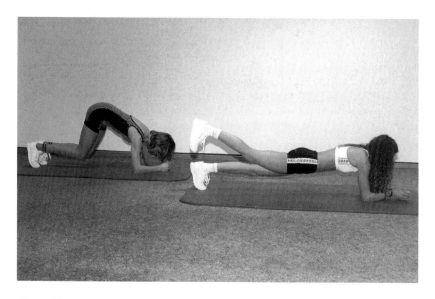

*Figure 33:*
*Exercise G25:Push-up position on lower arms lifting the legs alternately (left) –*
*variation (right)*

*b) Upper Thighs/Buttock*

## Exercise G26: Lifting the Leg from a Side Position
### (outside of thigh/abductor muscles)

**Execution:**       Lying on your side, the leg lying on top will be extended and lifted up. The lower one remains angled on the ground. Avoid bending the hip; the tip of the foot should be pulled forward to improve the tension of the body.

**Possible faults:**  The tip of the toe, not the heel points upwards.

**Variety:**         To make it easier, the other leg should be bent as well.

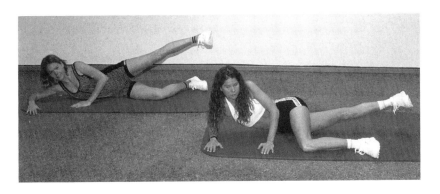

*Figure 34: Exercise G26: Lifting the leg from a side position (outside of thigh/abductor muscles) (left)*
*Exercise G27: Lifting the leg from a side position (inside of thigh/adductor muscles) (right)*

## Exercise G27: Lifting the Leg from a Side Position
### (inside of upper thigh/adductor muscles)

**Execution:**       You are in the same starting position as you were in the exercise before, only this time the lower leg gets a work-out. Bend the knee of the top upper leg and set the foot in front of the knee of the lower leg onto the ground. Now lift the stretched lower leg.

### Exercise G28: Lift the Leg while Sitting (front thigh)

**Execution:**        Sitting extended – one leg bend, foot on the ground, the stretched out leg will be lifted as high as possible.

**Variety:**        Lifting the leg while moving it to the side.

**Remark:**        Pull the tip of the foot of the extended leg towards you.

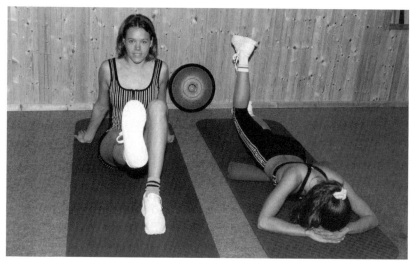

*Figure 35 Exercise G28: Lifting the leg while sitting (left)*
*Exercise G29: Lifting the leg while lying on one's belly (thigh, back, buttock) (right)*

### Exercise G29: Lift the Leg while Lying (thigh, back/buttock)

**Execution:**        While lying on your belly, move one leg upwards in a 90° angle, now push the sole of your foot upwards.

**Possible fault:**        Head in the neck

**Remark:**        This exercise will be good for your back if you prop a cushion or a rolled-up towel underneath your pelvis bone.

**Hint:**        The intensity of the specific leg exercises can be increased by using weight cuffs on the joints of your ankles.

### c) Shoulder Arm Musculature

## Exercise G30: Push-ups from the Knees (chest/back of upper arm)

**Execution:** Lying on one's belly, place the palms of hands next to your shoulders. The lower legs are angled upwards, the feet are crossed over each other. Now you take turns extending and bending the arms. *Important:* tension in the shoulder blade and stabilisation of the lumbar spine. When lowering yourself, inhale, exhale when pushing yourself up.

**Possible faults:** The lumbar vertebrae region is not supported sufficiently (it is "hanging through"), there will be an unfavourable strain on the intervertebral disc where the lumbar spine connects with the sacral bone.

**Variations:** When placing your hands further apart or placing them forward more you need a greater tension of the body. By putting your hands together more tightly you stronger exercise the upper arm and the chest muscles.

**Remark:** Push-ups on your knees is an excellent exercise if you still lack the strength to do the common push-ups. Often the common push-ups put an unphysiological strain on women because due to a lack of strength they cannot stabilise their shoulder blades sufficiently.

*Figure 36:*
*Exercise G30: Push-ups from the knees (left)*
*Exercise G31: One-armed push-ups (right)*

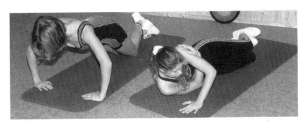

## Exercise G31: One-armed Push-ups

**Execution:** Lying on one side, you push up the upper body from the ground with the upper arm.

## 2.5 Strengthening with Small Equipment

### 2.5.1 Short Dumb-bells

### Exercise KH 32: Split Step (thigh, buttock)

**Execution:**    Take a step forward, then bend both knees until the knee in the back almost touches the ground. The knee up front has to stay over the joint of the foot.

**Possible faults:**    Round back, you do not push with the whole foot

**Variation:**    Put the short dumb-bells on your shoulders.

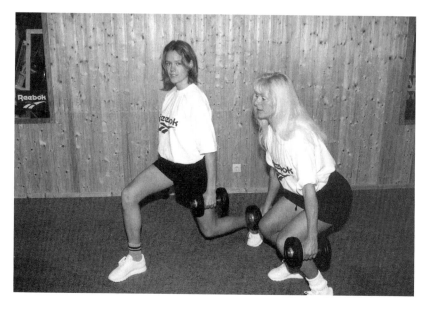

*Figure 37:*
*Exercise KH 32: Split step (it thighs/buttock) (left)*
*Exercise KH 33: Squats (it thighs/buttock) (right)*

## Exercise KH33: Squats (thighs/buttock)

**Execution:** The squat is without a doubt one of the best known exercises. The feet are shoulder width apart, the tips of the feet slightly point outwards. Slowly go down to a squatting position until the buttock is at the level of the knee. The whole foot remains on the ground. If this is not possible, the adductor muscles and the back of the leg are shortened. If this is the case, you should push a wedge underneath your heel. When stretching the back of the leg regularly, you will soon be able to do without the heel support and it will be easier to keep the back straight during the exercise.

**Possible faults:** Round back, knees do not remain in a straight line.

**Variation:** Put the short dumb-bells on the shoulders.

**Remark:** It is best for beginners to start with a quarter squat and increase their movement with growing security and body tension up to a half squat. Bending the knee a lot (angle between upper and lower thigh < 90°) should only be done in competitive sports.

## Exercise KH 34: Step Exercise (thigh, buttock)

**Execution:** Put your left foot on a bench or something like a bench and push yourself upwards by extending the hip and knee joint. The right foot is placed next to the left one. Slowly put the right foot on the ground again and repeat until getting fatigue. The movement should mainly come from the heel, not the ball of the foot because this would strain the knee too much.

**Variation:** Take turns putting the right and left foot in the back (easier).

*Figure 38:*
*Exercise KH34:*
*Step exercise (upper thigh, buttock) (left)*

*Exercise KH35: Lifting up front (shoulders/back) (right)*

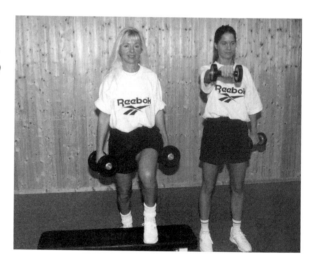

## Exercise KH 35: Frontal Lift (shoulders/back)

**Execution:** Take a short dumb-bell in each hand and hold them with almost straightened arms to the side of the body. Now you take turns moving the arms forward until they are in a horizontal position.

**Remark:** To avoid getting into a hollow back position, flex the belly and back muscles.

## Exercise KH 36: Side Lift (shoulder, neck)

**Execution:**      The almost extended arms are moved up sideways until they are in a horizontal position. The outer side of the hands point upwards during the whole exercise.

**Possible fault:**  Swing the weights up in the first third of the movement, turn of the hand in or outwards. Lifting higher than horizontal position.

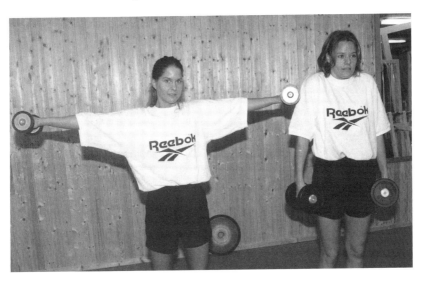

*Figure 39: Exercise KH36: Lifting sideways (shoulder/neck) (left)*
*Exercise KH37: Lifting the shoulder (neck, shoulder) (right)*

## Exercise KH37: Shoulder Lift (neck/shoulder)

**Execution:**       Take a dumb-bell in each hand and hold it with extended arms to the sides of the body. Now pick-up the shoulders until the throat has almost disappeared, then lower them again to the starting position. The arms remain straight.

**Possible faults:**  The shoulders fall down, bending the arms while lifting.

## Exercise KH38: Rowing (back)

**Execution:**    Standing position, feet are shoulder width apart, the knee joints are slightly angled, the upper body is bended forward while the hip is in an approx. 90° angle. The arms which are pointing downwards in the starting position are now evenly moved upwards.

**Possible faults:**    Head in the neck, movement of the trunk

**Variation:**    When not being able to stabilise enough, put one foot forward, use only one arm and support it with the other.

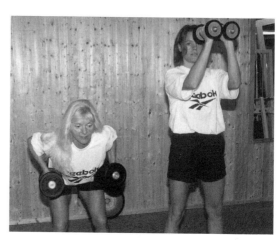

*Figure 40: Exercise KH38: Rowing (back) (left)*

*Exercise KH39: Butterfly (chest/shoulder) (right)*

## Exercise KH39: Butterfly (chest, shoulder)

**Execution:**    Standing position, the feet are shoulder width apart, the arms which are bent in a right angle are pulled up to the height of the shoulder. From this position lower the arms together in front of the face.

**Possible faults:**    Hollow back, shoulders are lifted

**Variation:**    Do the exercise while lying down, the lower arms are angled upwards, the elbows downwards. Imagine you are "hugging" a big ball.

**Remark:**    Especially slow execution of the exercise.

## 2.5.2 Therapeutic Band

### Exercise TB40: Powerwalking (upper thighs)

**Execution:** Tie up the band at the ends, if necessary repeatedly, "layer it" on top of each other so a ring of about 30cm diameter is made. Now slip the band over the ankles and stand straddle-legged to keep tension in the band. "March" on the spot moving the knees upwards and to the side. When placing the foot on the ground always roll it all the way to the heel.

**Possible faults:** Making a hollow back

**Variation:** Moving the heel in the back upwards and to the side.

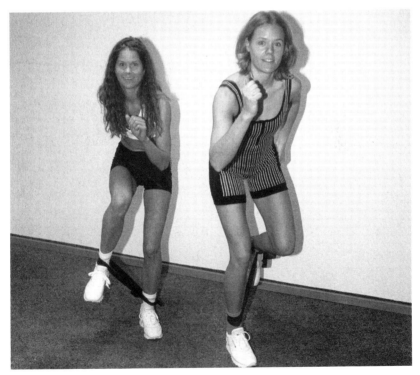

*Figure 41: Powerwalking (basic step with variations)*

## Exercise TB41: Leg Extension (buttock, hamstring)

**Execution:** We start in a bench position, the ends of the band are in your hands. The rubber band lies across the sole of the foot and can be wrapped around it once. Now you stretch the leg upwards without straightening the knee all the way.

**Possible faults:** Lack of trunk stability, making a hollow back

**Remark:** The intensity can quickly be adjusted by changing the position of the hand during the exercise.

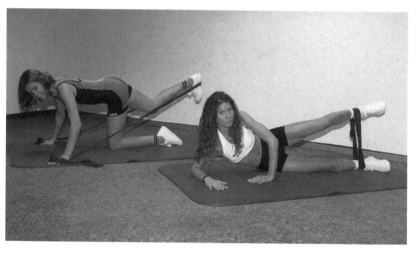

*Figure 42: Exercise TB41: Stretching the leg (buttock/hamstring) (left)*
*Exercise TB42: Straddling the leg away (buttock, abductor) (right)*

## Exercise TB42: Leg spread (buttock, abductors)

**Execution:** The knotted-up band is placed around the ankles, you are lying on your side. Lift the upper leg as much as possible and then slowly release.

**Remark:** If you have problems with the knees (lateral ligaments) you can also place the band around your knees.

## Exercise TB43: Kicks (front of the thighs)

**Execution:**      Tie the band up at a certain point (if possible below the height of the knees) and put it over the ankle of one leg. To begin pick the distance to the fixed point in a way that the band is slightly stretched. Now move the leg which is slightly flexed in the knee upwards and forwards.

**Variation:**      When turning 180° the hamstring is trained, turning 90° the inner/outer thigh is trained.

**Remark:**      To better stabilise the trunk you can use the back of a chair.

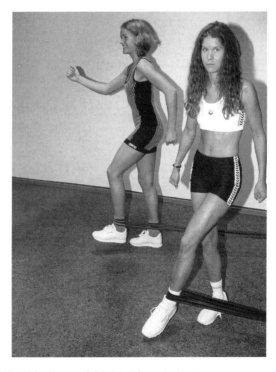

*Figure 43: Exercise TB43: Kicks (front of thigh/with variations)*

## Exercise TB 44: Rowing (upper back)

**Execution:** The middle part of the band is tied up, you hold the ends while sitting and then you move your arms, which are slightly angled at around shoulder height and backwards as much as possible.

**Variations:** The band can also be pushed diagonally upwards or downwards.

**Possible faults:** If the trunk is not stabilised it moves along when you do the rowing movement.

**Variations:** While performing the exercise the palms of the hands should be pointed up.

**Remark:** The intensity can be controlled by changing the distance to the fixed point.

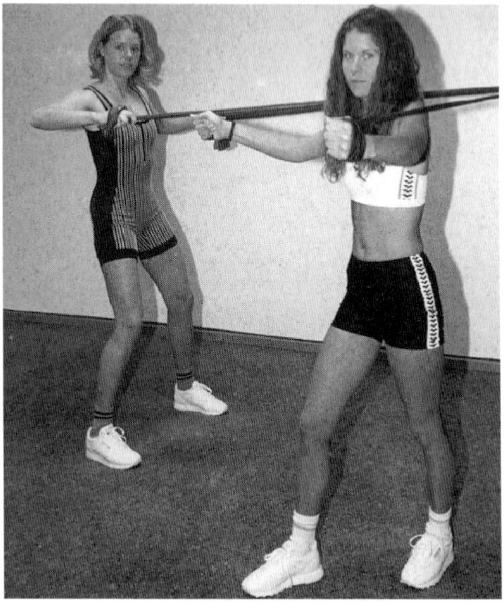

*Figure 44:*
*Exercise TB44: Rowing*
*(upper back) (left)*
*Exercise TB45: Butterfly*
*(chest) (right)*

## Exercise TB 45: Butterfly (chest)

**Execution:** The band is tied-up to a fixed point. You hold the ends. You pull your slightly bended arms together in front of the body.

## *Exercise TB 46: Pulling Sideways (shoulders)*

**Execution:**    You are in a step position, the front leg is placed onto the middle of the band the ends are wrapped around the hands. The slightly bent arms are moved up sideways until they are in a horizontal position.

**Variations:**    Raising the arms in a forward direction trains the front shoulder region

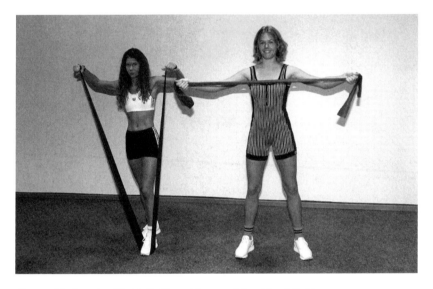

*Figure 45: Exercise TB 46: Pulling sideways (shoulders) (left)*
        *Exercise TB 47: Expander (upper back) (right)*

## *Exercise TB 47: Expander (upper back)*

**Execution:**    Sitting or standing spread leg, the ends of the band are wrapped around the hands, the arms extended to the front, the palms pointed up. Now move the hands at around the height of the chest to the side.

**Variation:**    Diagonal execution, meaning one arm will be moved slightly diagonally and up, the other slightly diagonally and down.

## Exercise TB 48: Triceps Muscle (back of the arm)

**Execution:**   Make a split step forwards. The opposite hand supports the band on the upper thigh, the elbow points backwards in a right angle. Stretch the arm out all the way to the back, the elbow remains stable as a turning point.

**Remark:**   If the band is very short between the grips, or if the band is folded together several times, the exercise is very intensive for the upper arm.

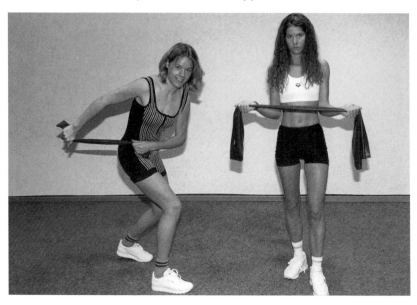

*Figure 46: Exercise TB48: Triceps muscle (back of the arm) (left)*
*Exercise TB49: Extension out the lower arm (shoulders)*

## Exercise TB49: Undercut Lower Arms (shoulders)

**Execution:**   The knees are slightly bent, the abdominal muscles are flexed. Both elbows press into the side of the body at a right angle, the palms of the hands are pointed up. Now slowly turn the lower arms outwards.

## Exercise TB50: „Lat-pull" (back/upper arm)

**Execution:** Standing position, legs closed hold the rubber band slightly tightened above your head. Now make a deep split step to the side while at the same time the corresponding arm is moved down and to the side; the other arm stays above the head.

**Remark:** Constantly switch sides during this work-out (right-left).

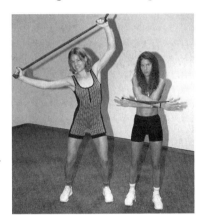

*Figure 47:*
*Exercise TB50: "Bib-pulling" (back/ upper arm) (left)*
*Exercise TB51: Folded arms (chest/upper arm) (right)*

## Exercise TB51: Arm crossing (chest/upper arm)

**Execution:** Standing up, your legs straddled apart, arms at the height of the chest. Now slowly cross the arms horizontally, tightening the band as intensive as possible.

**Remark:** Either after a few repetition, or after each you can lift the lower arm up without losing the tension in the band.

**Hint:** During all exercises with the expanding band it should be tight, even during the relaxing phases – never let it loosen up. It takes a little practise to tighten the band correctly in order to get the right diameter and hence the correct endurance span. Clips are available in special stores which enable a fast bow-making, and most of all they make the untying easier.

## 2.5.3 Pezziball or Fitball

### Exercise PB52: Strengthening of the Abdominals (straight abdominal musculature)

**Execution:** Lying with the back on top of the fit-ball, the shoulder girdle and head are lifted until they are horizontal, then they are slowly moved back into the starting position.

**Possible faults:** Overextension of the head and excessive outward curvature (kyphosis) of the thoracic spine should be avoided.

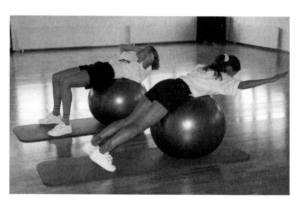

*Figure 48:*
*Exercise PB52:*
*Strengthening of the*
*abdominals(left)*

*Exercise PB53:*
*Extension of the trunk*
*(back/shoulder)*
*(right)*

### Exercise PB53: Stretching the Trunk (back/shoulder)

**Execution:** Arms, head and shoulder girdle are raised until in the final position the whole back from the tailbone to the back of the head is in a straight line with the arms extended. The movement should be made extremely slowly, almost in slow-motion.

**Possible faults:** The arms are used to get momentum, the head is pulled into the neck.

**Variations:** The arms are used to intensify the exercise. The closer to the trunk they are held the easier, and the farther they are extended the more difficult is the exercise.

## Exercise PB54: Leg Extension (buttock/back)

**Execution:** Lying on your belly, the legs are extended upwards and backwards until reaching a horizontal level. To improve the tension of the body it is more favourable to pull the tips of the feet towards the body.

**Possible faults:** A too low body tension, the head is pulled into the neck.

**Variations:** Dynamic performance, slowly alternating bending and extending of the legs.

*Figure 49:*
*Exercise PB54: Extending the leg (buttock/back) (left)*

*Exercise PB55: Standing up (thighs/buttock) (right)*

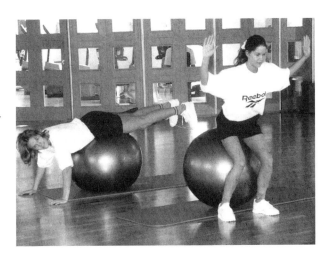

## Exercise PB55: Standing up (thighs/buttock)

**Execution:** Sit on the ball, bob up and down a little, then pick up the buttock a few centimetres while keeping the back straight. Try to stay in this position for as long as possible, then sit down again, bob up and down 3-4 times, repeat the exercise.

**Variation:** The arms can be crossed in front of the chest (easier) or extended out upwards (more difficult).

**Remark:** Only stand up so far that you still slightly touch the ball and it cannot roll away.

## Exercise PB56: Hip Lift (back/buttock)

**Execution:**      Lying on your back you place the lower legs onto the ball. The arms are lying to the side of the body, the inside of the palms point up. Flex the buttock muscles and back muscles and lift the pelvis until the body is extended all the way from the shoulder to the heel.

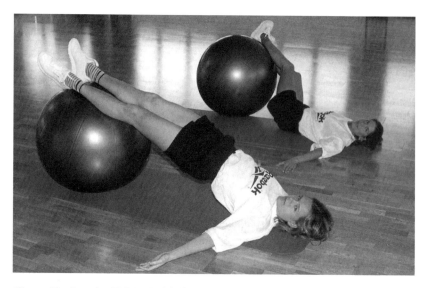

*Figure 50: Exercise PB56: Hip lift (back/buttock) (left)*
*Exercise PB57: Windshield-wiper (belly) (right)*

## Exercise PB57: Windshield-wiper (belly)

**Execution:**      Lying on your back, you put the lower legs onto the ball, the buttock very close to the ball. The arms lie next to the body, the inside of the hands press onto the ground. Roll the ball slowly to the right and to the left with your bent legs.

**Remark:**      The lumbar spine should not lose contact with the ground.

## 2.6 Work-out in a Fitness Centre

### Exercise F58: Abdominal Machine

**Execution:** By strongly flexing the abdominal muscles, the upper body will be bend forwards slightly. Lift the bended knees, combined with a small curl-up movement of the hip, improves the movement. At first it is difficult to keep the belly flexed while breathing at the same time.

**Possible faults:** Lack of tension in the abdominal muscles, making a hollow back. Pressing the feet too strongly onto the support.

**Variations:** By turning the upper body to the side, the slanted abdominal musculature is being worked on.

**Remark:** Due to some spine forms, for example if the spine is not able to bend a lot, problems in the lumbar vertebrae region can occur.

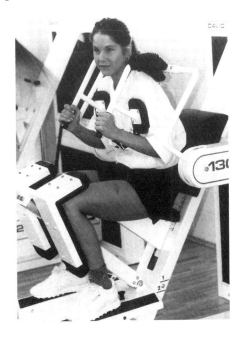

*Figure 51:*
*Exercise F58: Abdominal machine*

## Exercise F59:  Knee-lift with lower arm support
   *(Abdominals)*

**Execution:**  Press the lumbar region, not the upper back, against the support. Now when lifting the knee, the upper body can be bent forwards to get a full contraction of the abdominal muscles and only the lumbar vertebrae region is pressed against the support. Keep the hip angled when lowering the knee, the lift of the knees will be started by flexing the abdominal muscles.

**Remark:**  Often the exercise has to be stopped due to a lack of support in the muscles of the shoulders and arms. In this case you should practice the abdominal exercises explained in the previous chapters.

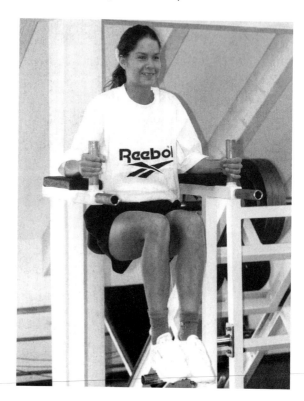

*Figure 52:*
*Exercise F59:*
*Knee-lift with lower*
*arm support*
*(Abdominals)*

## Exercise F60:   *Lifting the Knees while hanging (Abdominals)*

**Execution:**          While hanging on the rack, the knee is lifted higher than the hip – when lowering it, keep a small angle around the hip and introduce the pull-up movement by flexing the abdominal muscles.

**Possible faults:**    When hanging, the danger of overstretching is considerable. In this case, the first effort while lifting the legs comes from the lumbar region and the spine is at risk. Stretch the hip and the leg.

**Remark:**             This exercise can be executed well on wall-bars. Nevertheless, often the strength to hold oneself up is limited, meaning the arms will get tired before a big exercise effect is reached for the abdominals.

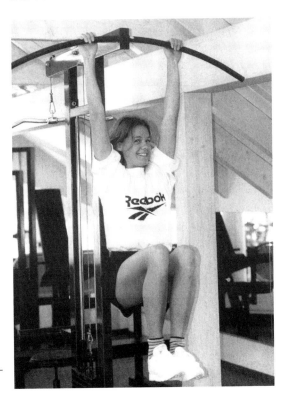

*Figure 53:*
*Exercise F60: Lifting*
*the knees while hang-*
*ing (Abdominals)*

## Exercise F61: Rotary Press

**Execution:** Sitting up straight, the pelvic bone is tipped forwards, you pull the resistance to the side and backwards while flexing the abdominal and the back muscles. No large movements. Especially during this exercise small, well-controlled movements should dominate.

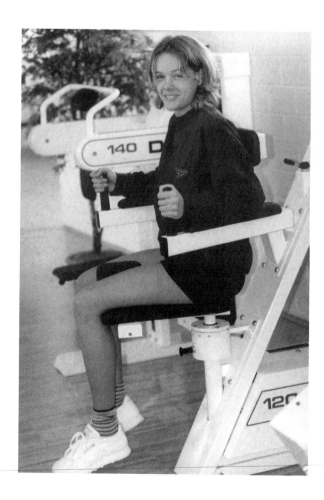

*Figure 54:*
*Exercise F61: Rotary press*

## Exercise F62: Bending Sideways at the Pulling Machine

**Execution:**     Stand uprigth and shoulder width apart and sideways to the pulling machine. Grab the grip with one
hand, put the other one on the neck. The arm holding
the grip is extended with the cable tight. Now bend
the upper body towards the machine and to the other
side against its resistance.

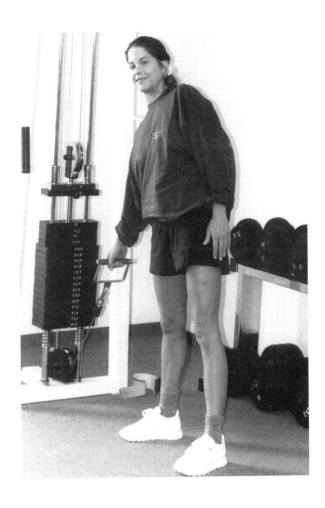

*Figure 55:*
*Exercise F62*
*Bending*
*sideways at the*
*pulling machine*

## Exercise F63: Sit-ups on the "Abdominal Bench"

**Execution:** on the back, the knees are bent, the upper body will be straightened just enough for the iliac crest to touch the board. The feet are fixed, the hands rest crossed in front of the chest or crossed behind the head to support it.

**Possible faults:** Fast and abrupt execution, the hands "pull" on the head. Your are pulling yourself up with the legs.

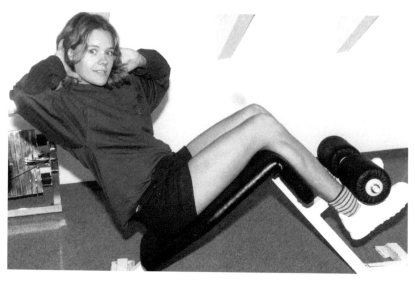

*Figure 56: Exercise F63: Sit-ups at the "abdominal bench"*

**Remarks:** Because the legs are fixed we actually have a false axis of rotation, meaning one mostly trains the shortened hip-flexors, therefore the straight muscle is loaded. In general, the straight abdominal muscle is only used during the first part of the straightening of the upper body. This movement more precisely is called the roll-up of the spine, during which the root and the beginning of the abdominal muscle are supposed to get closer to each other. The correct exercise instruction should be: "Push the costal arch in the direction of the 'bellybutton' and press the lumbar region tightly onto the support."

Recommendations: Views have changed over the years concerning posture and the effect of different exercises. Many people spend long enough in poor back posture today due to their sitting work position/life style, and because of this they should not assume the same position when exercising. The head should be held upright as an extension of the spine when lifting the shoulders girdle. One should look diagonally on the ceiling. A Lordoze-cushion is recommended to support the lumbar region, or perhaps a training bench with a cushion in-built. By that the abdominal muscles are trained from a pretensed position but just up to the horizontal position of the upper body.

During the mentioned sit-ups you can often notice that the person training will erect the upper body as stiff as a board and that while lowering it especially on the diagonal board or the "roman chair" which can be purchased everywhere right now, hollow back positions often occur which can put strong strains on the intervertebral ligament in the lumbar vertebrae region. The free swinging upper body makes out an arm of a lever which should not be underestimated. An additional risk are the arms when folded in the back. Often they are being used to get started. Due to this a faulty encumbrance as well as tension in the neck region can occur. Furthermore this position promotes the building of a hollow back during the exercise.

In addition to this, the "get-going motion" does not make any sense because the abdominal musculature should not be worked-out strong and fast.

In a lot of training centres, this problem tries to be decreased or evaded. Sit-ups will be performed with strongly bent knees which is very recommendable because in this position the hip is bent as well and the hip-flexor will not contract as much.

The second mentioned problem when doing this exercise, the endangerment of the intervertebral ligament due to avoiding the hollow back posture, multiplies on the diagonal board or "romain chair".

Therefore the people executing this exercise are urged to swing only with the upper body. In this way one can avoid making a swayback but a significant training of the straight abdominal muscles does not take place.

**Example:** Person A suffers from a strong swayback, a weak musculature of the abdominals and, resulting from this, a "paunch" (a forward arching belly). Person A often complains about backache. By all means A should train her abdominal muscles. Let's make her do the most suitable activities concerning these problems – sit-ups with legs being immobile.

The following can be noticed: At first the muscles to bend the hip, which is extremly shortened in people who have swaybacks, contract which puts a lot of tension onto the lumbar spine, meaning that at the very beginning of the movement already A has an excessive bridge-building in the lower back, the rump erects itself like a board, a bending of the spine cannot be noticed.

**Result:** This exercise shortens the hip-flexor even more. A is being pulled into a hyperlordosis even more, the tenseness in the back increases, hardly any training results on the abdominal muscles can be noticed. It is possible or even unavoidable that the backache gets worse.

## Exercise F64: Extensions

**Execution:**       Lay down flat on your belly onto the extension bench and slide forward with the upper body, the pelvis lies on the cushion, the lower thighs are fixed. Now slowly bend the upper body down and then lift it up again until it is in a horizontal position. The upward movement is started by flexing of the muscles of the buttock.

**Possible faults:** The head is pulled to the back, energetic execution of the exercise.

**Remark:**          Especially with people who suffer from hollow backs one can often notice that the head as well as the thoracic spine are in a horizontal position or even higher, while the lumbar spine is sagging. This can lead to back problems. If this is the case, the exercise should not be performed. The emphasis here lies on strengthening the abdominal muscles and the extension of the back extensors.

When crossing the hands behind the head, the result often is a round back in the thoracic vertebrae region. In this case it is better to cross the arms in front of the chest and to purposely push the elbows up and outwards when lifting the body into a horizontal position. This stabilises the shoulder blades and therefore prevents a round back.

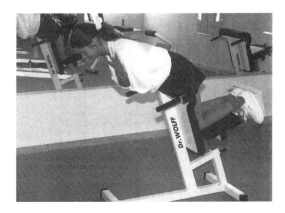

*Figure 57*
*Exercise F64: Extensions*

## Exercise F65: Stretching the Legs Backwards

**Execution:** Lie down on your belly up to about the hip bone (the hip joint stays mobile) onto the machine and support yourself at the sides with your hands. Now the legs are slowly moved until the body is horizontal. The tips of the feet pull towards the body.

**Possible faults:** Jerking, snappy lowering and stretching, head in the neck

**Variation:** The legs are alternately stretched (easier). The upper thigh, which is bent downwards, strongly presses against the box to stabilise the pelvis.

**Remark:** To increase the effect of the exercise, weight cuffs can be put around the ankles.

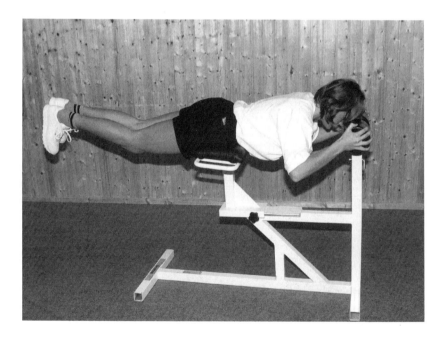

*Figure 58: Exercise F65: Stretching the leg backwards*

## Exercise F66: Butterfly Reverse

**Execution:** Press your upper body forwards against the cushion and the feet strongly onto the ground. Move the grips backwards in a half-circle. The elbows are slightly bent and stay at about the height of the shoulder during the whole movement.

**Possible faults:** The chest is not touching the cushion anymore, the shoulders are pulled up, vulture-neck.

**Remark:** Consciously try to move the shoulder blades.

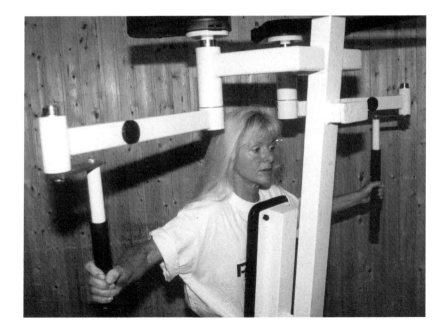

*Figure 59: Exercise F66: Butterfly reverse*

## Exercise F67: Neck Pull

**Execution:**   Grab the bar more than shoulder-width apart and sit down facing the machine. Immobilise your upper legs, the pelvis should be tipped forwards a little, the upper body should be straight and the head tipped forward a little. Now pull the bar in the direction of the neck, only so much that your elbows are pointing to the ground, meaning that no rotation in the shoulder girdle occurs.

**Possible faults:**   Lack of tension in the shoulder blades (can be recognised by a forward-hanging of the shoulder girdle)

**Remark:**   If there is a tendency towards developing a round back, the bar should be pulled down up front.

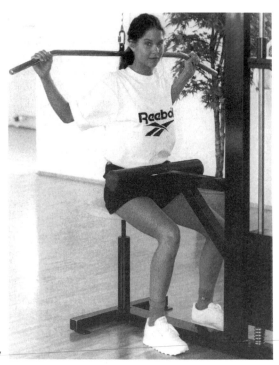

*Figure 60:*
*Exercise F67: Neck pull*

## Exercise F68: Back-extension Apparatus

**Execution:** Push the straight upper body backwards against the resistance of the roll, the knees remain angled. The distance between the arch of the ribs and the iliac crest has to always remain the same when pressing backwards as well as when moving forwards. The bending and extension is made in the joint of the hip, the back remains straight in itself as it should be during daily routine movements like stooping etc. Beginners should exercise with few repetitions only.

**Possible faults:** Extension of the upper thighs, the head pulled into the neck, sagging in the navel region

**Remark:** A mirror positioned to your side is ideal to check your posture.

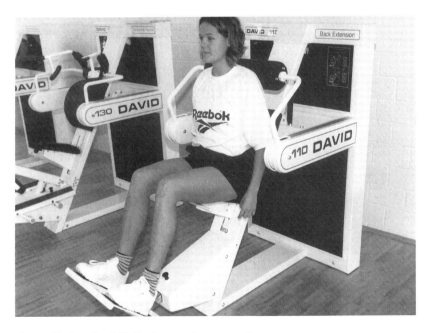

*Figure 61: Exercise F68: Back extension apparatus*

## Exercise F69: Rowing Machine

**Execution:** Pull the handles backwards, your upper body is erected – without the chest losing contact with the cushion. The feet press strongly onto the ground.

**Possible fault:** Round back, vulture neck

**Variation:** Change the grip on the handles, or the position of your elbows.

**Remark:** To get a better concentration on the back muscles only light weights should be used for the exercise. If the exercise is performed in a correct way and slowly, the shoulder blades open when pulling forwards, and when pulling back they get closer to each other.

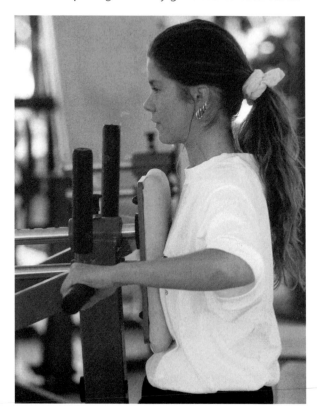

Figure 62:
Exercise F69:
Rowing machine

## Exercise F70:   Leg Extensor
### (front of thigh/stabilisation of the knee)

**Execution:**          The machine should be adjusted individually in accordance with the length of the upper and lower thigh. In order to do this an adjustable back support and a lower leg support which is adjustable in its height are needed. The joint of the knee should be at the height of the joint of the machine, if there is no gap between the hollow of the back of the knees and the cushion. You stretch the leg until it is horizontal, the point of the feet are pulled towards you.

**Possible faults:**    A too fast and too snappy extension and lowering

**Variation:**          If one leg was immobilised for a longer period of time (i.e. due to a plaster bandage) performing with only one leg can be an advantage when building-up the atrophied muscles again.

**Remark:**             If used for rehabilitative purposes, the machine should enable individual angles to start with, for example:
physician's recommendation: bend only 20°. The leg-extensor is not suitable for sports women who have problems with their cruciate ligaments. If the back of the knee caps (chondropathie patellae) shows signs of wear, the exercise should not be performed either.

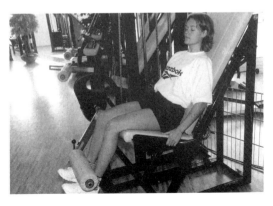

*Figure 63:*
*Exercise F70: Leg-extensor*

## Exercise F71: Knee Flexors (hamstrings)

**Execution:** Lying on your belly, the knee caps are not on the cushion, the roll is above your heels. Pay special attention that your buttock do not move up when bending your legs. If the support you are lying on is angled, a hyperlordosis is avoided. When lowering the legs you start another bending just before the legs are stretched out all the way.

**Possible faults:** A fast, uncontrolled lowering of the legs. Head pulled into the neck, making a hollow back.

**Remark:** Pick a low resistance which you can handle with the leg-flexor without making a hollow back.

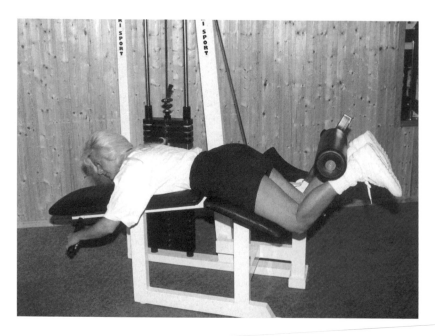

Figure 64: Exercise F71: Bending the legs

## Exercise F72: Leg-press (thighs/buttock)

**Execution:** While sitting the resistance will be pressed with the legs forward or diagonal upwards, depending on the machine. The feet should be hip-width apart. Point of the feet, knee and hip-bone form one line. Do not close the joints all the way when extending the legs and do not exceed a 90° angle between the upper and lower leg when bending your legs, otherwise the pressure-point of the knee-cap will be too great and there will be a risk of damaging the back of the knee cap. The back cannot be kept straight anymore when bending if the angle is bigger.

**Possible faults:** The knees make a movement inwards or outwards. The pressure is not built with all of the foot.

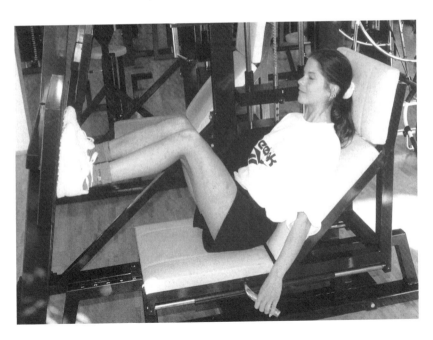

*Figure 65: Exercise F72: Leg-press*

## Exercise F73: Abductor Machine (thighs/buttock)

**Execution:** Spread your legs outwards, the pressure should be felt in the thighs to avoid a incorrect load of the knee joints.

**Remark:** Pay attention to an erect upper body. The significance of these muscles for the position of the pelvis, the bearing and the stabilisation of the leg, is always underestimated.

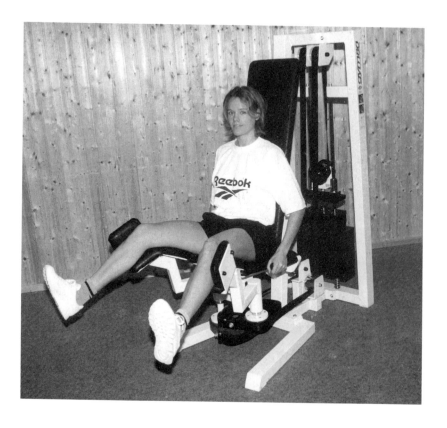

*Figure 66: Exercise F73: Abductor machine*

## Exercise F74: Adductor Machine (inside of thighs)

**Execution:** Pull your spread legs together, the pressure should be felt in the thighs to avoid a "scissor strain" in the joint of the knees.

**Remark:** As in exercise F73 pay attention to an erect upper body. Again the significance of these muscles for the position of the pelvis, the bearing and stabilisation of the leg is always underestimated.

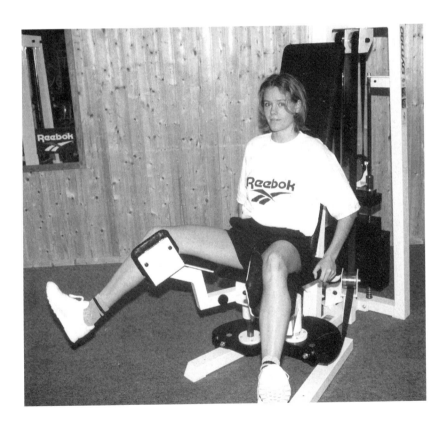

*Figure 67: Exercise F74: Adductor machine*

## Exercise F75: Hip extensor Machine (buttock)

**Execution:**   Adjust the machine to your height and lie down onto the bench with your upper body, the hip is not on the bench. Your left thigh presses against the support while your are extending your right leg against the resistance until it is in a horizontal position.

**Possible faults:**   Not extending the hip all the way

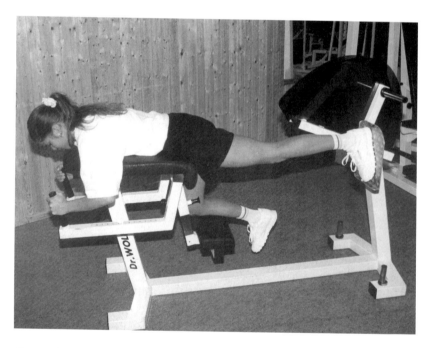

*Figure 68: Exersice F75: Glutaeus machine*

## Exercise F76: Cable Pull (buttock/thighs/lower back)

**Execution:** Stand facing the machine and fix the foot loop above the ankle. Bend your upper body forward far enough so the building of a hollow back can be avoided when moving the leg backwards.

**Possible faults:** Missing body tension. Evasive movement of the hips. The foot does not point downwards.

**Remark:** It is easier to perform this exercise if a weight disc is placed underneath the supporting leg.

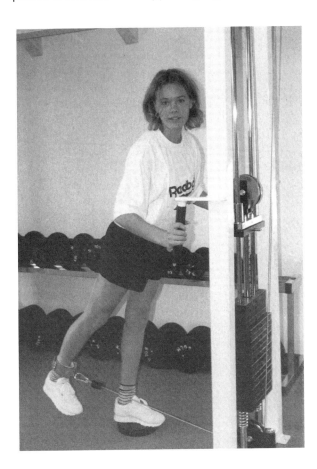

*Figure 69:*
*Exercise F76:*
*Cable pull*

## Exercise F77: Butterfly Machine (chest)

**Execution:** The feet are pressed strongly onto the ground, they are pressing the buttock and the back against the back support, the head also remains propped against the support extending the spine. The height of the seat has to be adjusted to get a right angle between the upper arms and the trunk. Press the cushions together just with the lower arms; the hands have a stabilising function.

**Remark:** Special attention has to be paid to the eccentric phase. Getting hurt due to overstrain can only be avoided by a slow and controlled backward movement of the cushions which can be done only by flexing of the muscles. A too frequent work-out on the butterfly machine can worsen your posture, it is important to combine this exercise with stretching exercises for the muscles (s. page 78) of the chest.

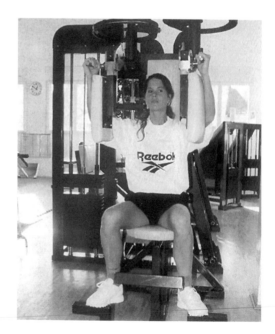

*Figure 70:*
*Exercise F77: But-*
*terfly machine*

## Exercise F78: Triceps Machine (arm-extensor/shoulder/neck)

**Execution:**  While standing, take the grips and press them down while sitting. Steady your thighs and sit in a straight position, meaning the pelvis is tipped forward, the shoulder blades are together, the breastbone is lifted up. Starting from this position you flex and extend the lower arms.

**Possible fault:**  Lifting the shoulders.

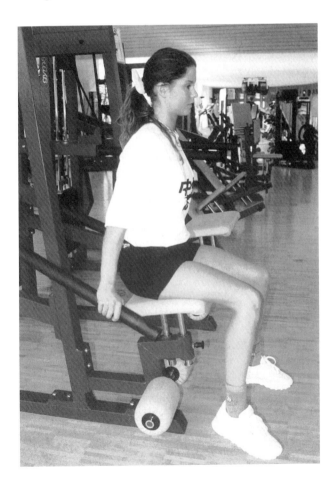

*Figure 71:*
*Exercise F78:*
*Triceps machine*

## 2.7 Relaxation

### Exercise E79: A Journey through Your Body

While lying on your back, close your mouth and start to control your breathing. Focus only on yourself and your body. Now imagine a small red dot which, starting in your right foot, slowly travels through all of your body. Always place yourself in that part of your body where dot is at the time and feel how heavy it is lying on the ground. A deep and calm inhaling and exhaling (abdominal breathing) supports the relaxing effect of this method. When done, stretch and extend like you do in the morning before getting up.

### Exercise F80: Breathing Relaxation

While lying on your back, place your hands onto your belly, close your eyes and feel the rising and falling of the abdominal wall in the rhythm of the breathing. When inhaling the abdominal wall lifts itself when exhaling it lowers. Time: 2-3 minutes calm deep puffs.

### Exercise E81: Relaxation according to Jacobsen

This method of progressive muscle relaxation works by systematically flexing and relaxing the muscle groups from head to toe. By doing so, a calming and relaxing effect on the body as well as on the soul is achieved. At first, the muscle is flexed and remains this way for 2-3 breaths, then relax and deeply exhale when doing so.

One has to concentrate strongly on the muscle, to be a part of it. A good sequence would be: right hand, lower and upper arm, then the left side, afterwards the muscles of the head and the face. For example: move eyebrows and nostrils, press the jawbones onto each other, continue with the neck, shoulders, abdomen, buttock, left upper and lower leg, right upper and lower leg.

A good thing to do is going to the sauna after participating in sport activities. The change between heat and cold strengthens your immune system and the circulation, and it is relaxing for the body, the spirit and the soul.

**Useful hints for a sauna visit:**

1. Be prepared to spend a lof of time there (about two hours).
2. Shower thoroughly. Dry yourself well afterwards - dry skin breaks into sweat faster.
3. Do not overdo it! Going to the sauna should not last longer than 12-15 minutes at about 90° (classic sauna temperature).
4. Before cooling off with cold plunges or under the shower, you should always go outside and take some deep breaths in the fresh air. Only use the diving or swimming-pool if you have taken a shower beforehand.
5. You should spend at least as much time well-covered in the relaxing room as you have in the sauna itself.
6. Going back into the sauna for a second or third time should be in accordance with the same procedures as before.
7. Drink a lot of mineral water.

# 2.8 Basics for a Health-oriented Muscle Training

- Avoid exercises involving a high or highest movement resistance since they bear the danger of overstraining, and the possibility of executing them badly.
- The economical movement of the extremities is only possible if the trunk is stable, extraneous movements are a result – especially when exercising close to the maximum capacity limit.
- Avoid exercises involving extreme positions of the body, like deep squatting, overstretching or bending forwards. Training which includes making a roundback or a hollow back, turning movements and the use of extra weights are not recommendable in any case.
- Avoid exercises which are performed at a high speed. Fast, jerky movements are less effective and cause injuries easier because the loading phase of the exercise is overcome by momentum. In particular the muscles of the trunk contain mostly slow reacting muscle fibres which take a long time to get tired and have to be worked on accordingly.

*Remember:* Calm and regularly instead of forcefully and abruptly!

• Pay attention to your breathing. Exhale when loading.

• Warm-up sufficiently before each work-out. It will protect you from getting injured, avoid long-term degenerative changes and improves your capacity.

• Stretch your muscles regularly, especially the parts which tend to shorten.

• Especially when doing strenuous work-out, make sure to take sufficient regeneration phases.

• Pay attention to an exact execution of the exercises. Often small things can make a big difference. Many exercises can be distinguished in easier or more difficult exercises by changing the grip. Rather pick the easier way to begin with and perform it correctly.

• Never exercise when it is causing you pain; never exercise over your threshold of pain.

• For health sports the dynamic strengthening with medium intensity should dominate.

## 2.9 Not like that – Unsuitable Exercises

It would be a little provocative to say that muscle training bears no dangers. Thinking that muscle training leads to a wear of the bones, the ligaments and joints however, is definitely not true. If health problems, injuries or late injuries occur, this always happens due to faults during training. Incorrectly picked-up or executed exercises always bear the risk of a bad strain or overstraining.

It is especially dangerous when work out close to one's limit because this often results in unavoidable movements of the trunk.

A further risk when doing muscle training is the overexercising of extremities. Correctly performed muscle training has to keep a main emphasis on the stabilisation of the trunk muscles, otherwise the spine is subject to even greater damage from the accelerated resistance by the arms.

This problem was explained in detail in the training part by using the individual exercises. When making a strong round back for example, the static strain on the intervertebral ligament in the region of the thoracic spine is increased by 50% compared to a normal formed back. Using a weight of 25 kg increases the vertical static strain on the 5. lumbar intervertebral ligament up to 480 kg while deep bending of the trunk with straight legs. You should also keep that in mind when grocery-shopping – a case of beer or juice weights about 20 kg.

When doing muscle training the weight should only be increased slowly, otherwise the result could be injuries due to overloading in the ligaments, tendons, joints and bones because the musculature will develop faster in this region than the ability to take load. A further important point about preventing injury when doing muscle training is keeping the body flexible. If you work-out a lot, the muscles shorten. This means it is easier to get hurt.

An improvement of the capacity is only possible anyway, if in addition to strengthening of the muscles, the movement capacity of the joint remains as it was or even improves.

We also have to mention the meaning of a good circulation. A pronounced capillarisation of the muscle fibres and a stable backflow of the veines is important. This means that, in addition to muscle training, regular endurance training for the stabilisation of the circulation is necessary as well.

A few "classical" examples of unsuitable exercises:

**Duck Walk**                    ***Negative effects***:

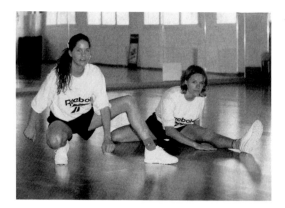

Strong overload of the knee-joints

*Figure 72: Duck walk (left)*
*Hurdle position (right)*

**Hurdle Bent**
***Negative effects:*** Because of the strong turning movement with bent knee-joints, the inner side ligament is overstretched and the inner meniscus overloaded.

**Plough**
**Negative effects:** Almost all of the bodyweight presses onto the neck and thoracic spine, therefore this region is being heavily overloaded.

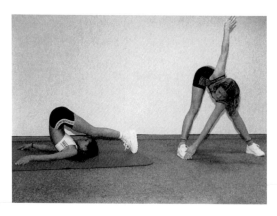

*Figure 73: Plough (left)*
*Diagonal turn of the trunk*
*(right)*

## Diagonal Turn of the Trunk
*Negative effects:* The turning of the spine leads to an anatomical load in the lumbar region.

## See-sawing on the Belly
*Negative effects:* Here an extreme hollow back position is developed overstraining the lumbar spine.

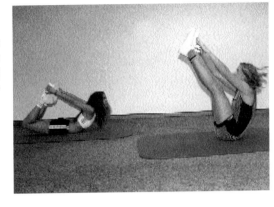

*Figure 74: See-sawing on the belly (left) Jack-knife (right)*

## Jack-knife
*Negative effects:* Especially if the musculature of the abdominals is weak, the lumbar spine is loaded too much, in addition to that it is not the abdominal musculature which is strengthened, but the already shortened hip-flexor.

## Pendulum of the Leg
*Negative effects:* Due to the long lever of the extended legs the spine is pulled into the hollow back and the lumbar spine is over-loaded.

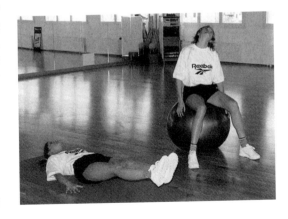

*Figure 75: Pendulum of the leg (left) Circling of the head (right)*

## Circling of the Head

*Negative effects:* The cervical spine is not a ball-joint (as for example the shoulder blade is) and therefore not meant to do circling movements. Uncontrolled and fast movements additionally load the cervical spine strongly and anatomically.

## Circling of the Trunk

*Negative effects:* The spine is not made to do powerfull circling movements. Also looking at it from a training benefit, there is no plausible reason for this exercise, therefore it should not be performed.

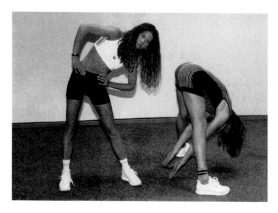

*Figure 76:*
*Circling of the trunk (left)*
*Forward bending from the*
*trunk (right)*

## One-sided Bending forward of the Trunk

*Negative effect:* This strong bending overloads the lumbar spine.

# 3 Programmes

What follows is the introduction of some programmes which should enable you to turn the advice you just read in this book into action.

The programmes were put together in a way so that they can be performed without or with very little equipment in your own home or in a training room with equipment.

For some of the exercises you will need – in addition to a comfortable mat for the exercises you perform on the ground, an exercise ball, an expanding exercise band or short dumb-bells, all inexpensive equipment.

A lot of the described exercises can be intensified by putting weight cuffs on the hand joints and ankles. But basically increasing the number of repetitions is sufficient to increase the training effect.

If you own equipment such as a home-trainer or a mini-trampoline, make use of these when warming-up or during the endurance training.

**Music:**
It is a well-known fact, that music makes it all go easier. Pick out your music, the rhythm of it can be used as an orientation help but do not force yourself to do every exercise in the rhythm of the beat. The exact choice of the music which beat exactly reflects the rhythm of the exercise is a science by itself.

The music has to meet your personal taste and motivate you to move. For stretching exercises and the relaxing part use calm, instrumental music.

## 3.1 Beginners All-round Home Programme

### 3.1.1 Without Equipment

| Training part | Exercise |
|---|---|
| **Warm-up** | 1. A3:  Running while shadow-boxing<br>2. S6:  Calf<br>3. S5:  Back of thigh<br>4. S9:  Front of thigh<br>5. S13: Chest/shoulder<br>6. S11: Lower back |
| **Main part** | 7. G16: Abdominal straight<br>8. G30: Push-ups on the knees<br>9. G26: Lifting up the leg while lying on the side<br>10. G27: Lifting up the leg while lying on the side<br>11. G28: Lifting the leg while sitting<br>12. G21: Diagonal arm-leg-lifting<br>13. G18: Pressing the knee |
| **Cool down** | 14: E80: Breathing relaxation |

### 3.1.2 With the Pezziball

| Training part | Exercise |
|---|---|
| **Warm-up** | Exercises 1-6 as in programme 3.1.1 |
| **Main part** | 7. PB52: Strengthening of the abdominal<br>8. PB53: Stretching the trunk<br>9. PB56: Lifting the hip<br>10. PB57: Windshield-wiper<br>11. PB55: Standing up |
| **Cool down** | 12. E80:  Breathing relaxation |

# 3.2 Advanced All-round Home Programme

## 3.2.1 Without Equipment

| Training part | Exercise |
|---|---|
| **Warm-up** | 1. A3:  Running while shadow-boxing<br>2. A2:  Jumping to the side<br>3. S6:  Calf<br>4. S5:  Back of thigh<br>5. S9:  Front of thigh<br>6. S13: Chest/shoulder<br>7. S11: Lower back |
| **Main part** | 8. G16: Abdominals straight<br>9. G20: Lifting of the pelvis<br>10. G19: Lifting the leg while lying on the side<br>11. G22: Alternately lifting shoulder/leg<br>12. G24: Lifting the trunk while kneeling<br>13. G29: Lifting the leg while lying on the belly<br>14. G30: Push-ups from the knees<br>15. G26: Lifting the leg while lying on the side<br>16. G27: Lifting the leg while lying on the side |
| **Cool down** | 17. S8:  Adductor<br>18. S7:  Adductor<br>19. E81: Relaxing according to Jacobsen |

## 3.2.2 With Short Dumb-bellts

| Training part | Exercise |
|---|---|
| **Warm-up** | Exercises as in programme 3.2.1 |
| **Main part** | 8. KH32: Split step<br>9. KH38: Rowing<br>10. KH 39: Butterfly |

11. KH34:  Step exercise
12. G17:    Diagonal crunches
13. G20:    Lifting of the pelvis
14. KH36: Lifting of the side
15. KH37: Lifting up the shoulders

**Cool down**          16. S13: Chest/shoulder
17. E81: Relaxing according to Jacobsen

### 3.2.3 Short Programme – Strengthening with the Therapeutic Band

| **Training part** | Exercise |
|---|---|
| **Warm-up** | 1. A4:      Diagonal knee and elbow |
| | 2. TB40:  Powerwalking |
| **Main part** | 3. TB41: Stretching of the leg |
| | 4. TB42: Spread the leg up |
| | 5. TB44: Rowing |
| | 6. TB45: Butterfly |
| | 7. G20:   Lifting of the pelvis |
| | 8. TB46: Pulling sideways |
| | 9. TB50: Bib-pulling |
| **Cool down** | 10. S5:   Back of thigh |
| | 11. S9:   Front of thigh |
| | 12. S13: Chest/shoulder |
| | 13. S11: Lower back |

# 3.3 Training in a Fitness Centre

| Training part | Exercise |
|---|---|
| | |

**Warm-up**
1. A1:  Bike ergometer/stepper
2. S6:  Calf
3. S5:  Back of thigh
4. S10: Bending the hip
5. S13: Chest/shoulder
6. S11: Lower back

**Main part**
7. F69: Rowing machine
8. F72: Leg-press
9. F59: Knee-lift with lower arm support
10. F73: Abductor machine
11. F74: Adductor machine
12. F61: Rotary Press
13. F77: Butterfly machine
14. F66: Butterfly revers
15. F58: Abdominal machine
16. F68: Back-stretching apparatus

**Cool down**
17. A1:  Bike ergometer/stepper

# 3.4. Programmes Emphasising Certain Body Parts

## 3.4.1 Shoulder-neck-region

| Training part | Exercise |
|---|---|
| **Warm-up** | 1. A4: Diagonal knee and elbow |
| | 2. A3: Running while shadow-boxing |
| **Main part** | 3. G21: Diagonal arm-leg-lifting |
| | 4. KH37: Lifting up the shoulder |
| | 5. KH36: Sideways lifting |
| | 6. KH35: up front |
| | 7. KH38: Rowing |
| **cCool down** | 8. S13: Chest/shoulder |
| | 9. S14: Back of the neck area |
| | 10. S15: Side of the neck |
| | 11. S11: Lower back |
| | 12. E79: Journey through the body |

## 3.4.2 Back

| Training part | Exercise |
|---|---|
| **Warm-up** | 1. A3: Running while shadow-boxing |
| | 2. S5: Back of thigh |
| | 3. S9: of thigh |
| | 4. S13: Chest/shoulder |
| **Main part** | 5. G21: Diagonal arm-/leg-lifting |
| | 6. G19: Lifting the leg while lying on the side |
| | 7. G22: Alternatively lifting shoulder/leg |
| | 8. G23: Lifting the pelvis |
| | 9. G24: Lifting the trunk while kneeling |
| | 10. G25: Push-up position on lower arms lifting legs belly |
| **Cool down** | 11. S10: Bending the hip |
| | 12. S11: Lower back |

## 3.4.3 Upper Thigh and Buttock

| Training part | Exercise |
|---|---|
| **Warm-up** | 1. A3:   Running while shadow-boxing<br>2. TB40: Powerwalking |
| **Main part:** | 3. TB41: Stretching the leg<br>4. TB42: Stretching the leg sideways<br>5. G28:  Lifting the leg while sitting<br>6. G29:  Lifting the leg while lying on the belly<br>7. G19:  Lifting the leg while lying on the side<br>8. G23:  Lifting the pelvis<br>9. TB43: Kicks (with all variations) |
| **Cool-down** | 10. S5:  Back of thigh<br>11. S7:  Abductors-muscles<br>12. S8:  Adductors-muscles<br>13. S10: Bending the hip |

## 3.4.4 Stomach

| Training part | Exercise |
|---|---|
| **Warm-up** | 1. A4:   Diagonal knee and elbow<br>2. A11:  Lower back<br>3. S10:  Bending the hip |
| **Main part** | 4. G16: Stomach straight<br>5. G17: Diagonal crunches<br>6. G22: Alternatively lifting shoulders/legs<br>7. G19: Lifting the leg while lying on the side<br>8. G20: Lifting up the pelvis<br>9. G25: Push-up position on lower arms<br>          lifting legs belly |
| **Cool down** | 10. E80: Breathing relaxation |

# APPENDIX

# Bibliography

BÖS, K.: Fitness testen und trainieren. München 1996.

BRÜGGER, A.: Gesunde Körperhaltung im Alltag. Zürich 1989.

EHLENZ, H. u.a.: Krafttraining. München 1991.

ENGELHARDT, M.: Sportmedizin. München 1994.

FREIWALD, J.: Prävention und Rehabilitation im Sport. Reinbek 1989.

FREIWALD, J.: Aufwärmen im Sport. Reinbek 1991.

GROSSER, M. u.a.: Richtig Muskeltraining. München 1987.

GUNNARI, u.a.: Allround Fitness. Reinbek 1989.

HAMM, M.: Fitness Ernährung. Hamburg 1990.

HOLLMANN, W.: Sportmedizin. Stuttgart 1990.

HOLLMANN, W.: Prävention und Rehabilitation von Herz-Kreislaufer-
krankungen durch körperliches Training. Stuttgart 1983.

KEMPF, H.D.: Die Rückenschule. Reinbek 1990.

KNEBEL, K.: Funktionsgymnastik. Reinbek 1985.

KOMI, P.V. (HRSG.): Kraft und Schnellkraft im Sport. Köln 1994.

KONOPKA, P.: Sporternährung. München 1994.

KREUZRIEGLER, F. u.a.: Anti-Osteoporose-Training. Oberhaching 1991.

LAGERSTRÖM, D.: Freizeitsport. Erlangen 1983.

MARTIN, D.: Handbuch der Trainingslehre. Schorndorf 1991.

MÜLLER-WOHLFAHRT, H.-W. u.a.: Verletzt ... was tun? Pfaffenweiler 1996.

OW VON, D.: Muskuläre Rehabilitation. Erlangen 1987.

REINHARDT, B.: Gesunder Rücken – Besser Leben. Erlangen 1989.

ROST, R.: Herz und Sport. Erlangen 1991.

SÖLVEBORN, S.: Stretching. München 1983.

TERRY, P.: Mental zum Sieg. München 1990.

UNGER, E.: Handbuch für Muskeltraining. Aachen 1995.

WEINECK, J.: Optimales Training. Erlangen 1987.

WOLFF, H.: Präventivmedizinisch orientiertes Fitnesstraining. Erlensee 1990.